Facing Facial Pain

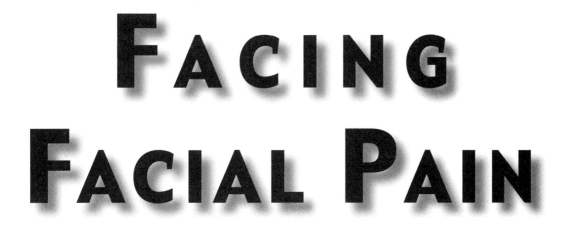

FACING FACIAL PAIN

Your Role in
Ending the Pain

GERALD M. LEMOLE, MD
EMILY JANE LEMOLE, MA

FOREWORD BY DR. OZ

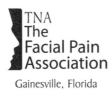

TNA
The
Facial Pain
Association
Gainesville, Florida

Facing Facial Pain: Your Role in Ending the Pain

Printed in the United States of America

Worldwide distribution by Collage Books Inc.

ISBN: 978-0-9672393-6-1

First Printing

Published by

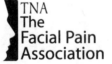

TNA
The
Facial Pain
Association

408 W. University Ave., Suite 602, Gainesville, FL 32601

10   9   8   7   6   5   4   3   2   1

Dedicated to
Gwen McQueen Asplundh
And to
TNA/The Facial Pain Association

CONTENTS

PART ONE: THE FACIAL PAIN PUZZLE

PART TWO: THE LEMOLE
RECOVERY PROGRAM

PART THREE: THE NUTRITION AND SCIENCE OF FACIAL PAIN

ACKNOWLEDGMENTS

The authors offer their thanks and gratitude to several people who have together shepherded this book along from conception to completion:

Michael Pasternak first invited us to present our healing approach to facial pain at the national conference in 2000 of what was then called the Trigeminal Neuralgia Association – now TNA/The Facial Pain Association. Patients who attended that conference (and later ones) strongly encouraged us to "write the book." Michael, then TNA's conference coordinator and eventually its president, developed a profound interest in finding ways to eliminate the suffering of people with facial pain through innovative approaches to alternative and complementary medicine. He functioned as foreman of this project, keeping all of us moving toward the goal: "Write the book."

Mike Hirsch, a long-time member of the Board of Directors of TNA – and another past president – encouraged us to convert some preliminary spiral-bound notes into an expanded vision that ultimately became *Facing Facial Pain*. His continuous support over nearly a decade since that first meeting was absolutely key to our completing this project.

Doris Odhner Delaney not only "key-stroked" every word of our manuscript (and our handwritten notes and phone messages and audio tapes), but she routinely helped us find the precise word to help express an idea. She researched and fact-checked tirelessly, organized hundreds of interrelated and overlapping segments of text and graphics, and assembled the final manuscript.

Richard Marschner, besides being a member of the TNA/ The Facial Pain Association board of directors, is a skilled and patient wordsmith who has helped transform a rough manuscript into a book of which we are all very proud. We are grateful for the wonderful way Rich has worked as our editor at the nerve center of our team. He and Doris functioned as a remarkably effective team without whose endless contributions our overall vision could never have been accomplished.

Gwen Asplundh, who provided the inspiration for this book, deserves our special thanks.

FOREWORD

John Fothergill gave the first full and accurate description of trigeminal neuralgia in 1773, but earlier descriptions of TN (Fothergill's disease) can be inferred from the writings of Galen in Asia Minor two thousand years ago and in the 11th century by Avicenna, who called TN "tortura oris." Undoubtedly, some images depicting "toothache" suffers from remote eras actually represented patients with this ailment, since dental caries were uncommon until modern times.

So why has such an ancient malady remained uncured in a time where modern medicine has made remarkable advances in understanding the molecular mechanisms of diseases and offering high tech solutions? This is the challenge that Dr. Gerald Lemole embarks upon with this wonderful summary of trigeminal neuralgia -- the ailment, its causes, and its potential treatments. What makes this "owner's manual" for trigeminal neuralgia so valuable is its comprehensive holistic approach to treating a chronic illness that has multiple avenues of recovery and relapse.

Although he's an internationally renowned cardiac surgeon, Dr. Lemole would not be the most likely candidate to create a book that will serve many trigeminal neuralgia sufferers, their families and their caregivers so admirably. He does not have the ailment himself. He has not specialized in neurologic ailments in the past. But over the course of 40 years as a healer, Dr. Lemole began identifying fundamental, recurrent problems that cause many of the chronic illnesses that afflict so many Americans.

The inflammation that precipitates heart disease is also an underlying problem in many neurologic conditions. Think of inflammation as the rusting of our bodies, accelerated by oxidation and other natural processes that usually are naturally kept in check. For example, when you cut an apple in half, the browning process that ensues over 20 minutes is caused by oxidation. Squeezing a lemon over the half apple will retard the color change because lemon juice contains the anti-oxidant vitamin C. When we consume vitamin C, we also slow the oxidation process within our bodies.

Abnormally functioning regulatory processes like inflammation and oxidation are worsened by toxins and by the inability of our lymphatic systems to support a dysfunctional immune system that mistakenly begins to bring "friendly fire" onto our own tissues. Lymphatics are particularly interesting because most of us know little of this essential system of waste removal from the body. Your lymph nodes are the lumps that form in your neck when you get a sore throat. They connect the lymph channels throughout the body, and their tiny muscles "milk" the fluid back toward your heart when you are active. Massage will stimulate lymph drainage as well, which may explain why a massage is so soothing – and is such a darn good idea.

Once we understand the basics regarding trigeminal neuralgia, we can launch into the recovery program designed by Dr. Lemole. To explain the fundaments, please allow me a brief autobiographical segue.

I made the smartest decision of my life 25 years ago by marrying Dr. Lemole's eldest daughter Lisa. At the time, I was a traditional medical student, studying pharmacology and physiology with our conventional textbooks and memorizing established rules for treating illness. On my first visit to his home, I was struck by the remarkable insight that the Lemole family had somehow bottled "wellness". The six children looked and behaved healthily. The secret seemed to be that Mrs. Lemole had created a sanctuary for healthy living, including herb gardens, a vegetarian lifestyle and an appropriate skepticism of long-established medical rules.

Dr. Lemole was already famous for developing numerous innovative solutions in treating advanced heart disease surgically. After graduating from Temple University medical school, he was trained at the remarkable Baylor cardiac surgical training program in Houston with Drs. DeBakey and Cooley. Dr. Lemole participated in the first human heart transplant in the country, then returned to the Northeast as the youngest chief of cardiac surgery ever. He performed the first coronary artery bypass in the area and invented devices to repair torn aortas and complete other complex operative procedures. His many contributions to the field earned him numerous academic accolades, including membership in the most prestigious heart-surgery societies.

Despite all these successes within conventional medicine, Dr. Lemole was increasingly open-minded to innovative healing approaches. Once while playing a heated game of Trivial Pursuit with the family, I was stumped by the question, "Which famous surgeon earned the nick name 'Rock-a-doc' by being the first to play rock music in the operating room". My father-in-law won the point -- and game -- by offering his own name. Dr. Lemole had permitted the playing of music in his operating theatre in order to help the team and patient relax so all could participate most effectively. He brought this same openness to alternative and complementary healing approaches.

Throughout my adult life, I have enjoyed enormously watching Dr. and Mrs. Lemole (AKA my "in-laws") battle over the best path for healing friends and family. One discussion surrounded their sister-in-law Gwen, who was suffering from trigeminal neuralgia with no clear course of treatment yet identified within conventional medicine. Over the course of several months, the Lemoles offered solutions that dramatically reduced Gwen's symptoms of TN, and the experience awakened the sleeping giant of an idea. Could *many* of our chronic illnesses be treated with a simple recovery program which we know is effective in other well-studied ailments like atherosclerotic heart disease and certain cancers?

This brings me back to the Lemole Recovery Program, which is the heart and soul of this book.

We must understand that when we walk into a grocery store, we are really walking into a pharmacy. The powerful nutrients found in colorful vegetables and fruits were created to protect these products from the sun and other oxidizing stimuli. We share these healing nutrients by consuming this produce. The Lemole Food Pyramid outlines this insight elegantly and offers a logistically simple pathway to making the correct food choices. Adding the micronutrients and herbs described to the mix reinforces the healing power of food. As a side benefit, you get to lose weight effortlessly with the 14-day diet plan, supported by the many recipes in chapter 10. Adding effective management of the stress of modern life, and doing smart exercises -- including the aforementioned massage -- helps keep the immune system functioning at full speed and playing for the right team -- *yours!*

Part III of this comprehensive survey helps all of us understand the underlying science behind many of Dr. Lemole's insights, and much of this material will be of more importance to your healers than to you -- orthomolecular medicine, vitamin D science, antioxidant details, the myths of cholesterol, and the deeper insights that explain healthy aging. Why is this foundation of science included in a book designed for patients and their loved ones? All too often, ground-changing books like this sit on a patient's bookshelf without ever being digested by the doctors and nurses who treat trigeminal neuralgia.

The one request that I have for each reader of this book is that they share Part III with their healers so we can all spread the word. You are now in the army that will carry this banner for a smart treatment approach that actually can help those suffering from trigeminal neuralgia. By being one of the bumble bees that fertilizes the pods of learning from which your healers feed, you are helping modern medicine treat this and other chronic illness.

Bless you for doing this, despite your own suffering.

Mehmet Oz, M.D.
Host, "The Dr. Oz Show"
Professor and Vice Chair, Department of Surgery,
Columbia University/New York Presbyterian
Medical Center

INTRODUCTION

The Lemole Recovery Program for Trigeminal Neuralgia and Related Facial Pain

Much of what follows is taken from the introduction to my 2001 book, *The Healing Diet – A Total Health Program to Purify Your Lymph System and Reduce the Risk of Heart Disease, Arthritis, and Cancer.* It remains as true today as it was then, and it helps explain why we decided to write this second book in an effort to help patients with trigeminal neuralgia and other facial pain manage their condition and regain their health.

I am a heart surgeon. I am only one among hundreds of specialists qualified to perform these complicated, sophisticated and life-saving procedures. Over the course of my cardiovascular surgery career, I have been responsible for more than 20,000 such operations. In hospitals world-wide, lives are saved because we've built new routes in the body for blood to reach the heart, or installed a machine to keep a heart pumping, or substituted one heart for another. No one – with the possible exception of the patients and their loved ones – thinks that anything particularly out of the ordinary has occurred. They expect us to save lives. That's what cardiac surgeons are for.

For as long as I can remember, I wanted to be a doctor. My father owned a pharmacy on Staten Island and he, my mother, my two brothers and I lived in an apartment upstairs. Quite naturally, doctors were among my father's closest friends, and several played in his weekly card games. I grew up to wonderful stories of live-saving operations and dramatic emergency procedures performed by these community heroes and family friends.

While studying to become a general surgeon, I attended a lecture at Temple University by Dr. Michael DeBakey, the pioneer of human heart-transplant surgery – and later, lung-transplant surgery. In 1967, I went to Houston to study with his team. Heart surgery was very new, very challenging, and very exciting. My colleagues and I were truly astronauts of medical science, walking on terrain where no one else had ever been.

From then on, the development of my professional career was relatively straightforward. The heart became the abiding interest in my life. I decided to concentrate not only on transplants and bypass surgery, but on operations that were often simpler, though no less live-giving. Because we were having trouble with heart transplants – too often, patients' bodies rejected them, leaving no hope for their survival – I wanted to find ways to make heart operations safer and more reliable.

In 1969, I returned to Temple University to become an instructor in surgery, and soon was named chief of cardiothoracic surgery. The same year, I performed the first coronary bypass in that part of the country. Over the next few years, I became a full professor at Temple and was named chief of surgery at Deborah Heart and Lung Center in Browns Mills, NJ – all the while continuing my other duties at Temple. In 1986, I was asked to become head of cardiac surgery at the Medical Center of Delaware – now the Christiana Health Care System – a job I held for more than 20 years.

I consider myself a good scientist – a surgeon who has mastered both his craft and the medical machinery that has made it easier to do it well. I am very much a part of the "medical establishment." But along the way, several things have happened to broaden my view. Now, I view surgery and its attendant medical equipment as only one part of the overall treatment for heart disease. I have become as interested in disease prevention as I am in cure. I have become aware that diet, exercise, stress management and an abundance of spirituality – yes, spirituality – are all essential to maintaining a sound heart. And I have also become aware of the crucial role played by a healthy lymphatic system – that miraculous network of pipes and nodes that serves as the body's cleansing system – not only in maintain heart health, but in avoiding a wide variety of chronic conditions. This is what convinced me to write *The Healing Diet* in 2001.

What lead to Janie's and my awareness of how all this may apply to the treatment of facial pain and other nerve conditions – and our decision to write this second book – is a decades-long story; here is a *very* short version.

❖ ❖ ❖ ❖ ❖

When I was a freshman in medical school, I met a beautiful young woman named Emily Jane Asplundh, then in her first year as an undergraduate. We dated a few times but soon separated – I was a traditional Roman Catholic; she was a Swedenborgian. Our theological arguments – I recall one in particular about the nature of evil – were what I remembered most about those few dates. When we met again three years later, we began to date seriously, and in seven months we were married.

After I started my residency, Janie began going through my medical journals, clipping articles she thought would interest me. In effect, the process introduced her to medicine, and gradually she expanded her reading – and clipping – to books and periodical articles about the healing power of certain foods and herbs. Later, her reading focused on the healing effects of stress management and spirituality. This was long before the concept of mind-body medicine had reached the American consciousness – and I was definitely one of the skeptical scientists who discounted most of it.

But I *didn't* discount Janie's ideas. She wasn't a flower child or a kook. I knew her spirituality came from a deep commitment to God, and her focus on diet came from what had been years of study in the area of nutrition and holistic health. Yet while I trusted her intuition, I thought she was uneducated in science and medicine.

"You don't understand what doctors do," I said.

"Doctors don't have training in health, diet or nutrition," she countered.

She knew that American doctors are taught strictly pharmacological medicine – our quick-fix prescriptive approach. We're used to hearing our patients say, "Help me; give me a pill to make me feel better." But too often, this is the wrong approach. It concentrates on the elimination of symptoms, not the cause of the problem.

"The hard work of changing lifestyle and diet can make an enormous change in people's lives," Janie later told a reporter. "It isn't a substitute for medicine – it complements medicine. Much of being healthy is a choice."

I had to agree with her. In my four years in medical school, and throughout my residency, I could count on one hand the number of lectures on nutrition. These basic sessions focused on the importance of "a well-balanced diet," but such a traditional and old-fashioned view of a balanced diet had by that time become, in fact, dangerously out of date.

My conversion to Janie's way of thinking came slowly. But when the connection between diet and the lymphatic system became clear to me, I decided I'd try Janie's regimen on my heart patients. Maybe vitamins and herbs, vegetables and fruits would help clear the lymphatic system. Maybe – just maybe – such a program could reduce the risk of a second heart attack.

So in about 1980, while the medical establishment continued to scoff at "the health-food fad" endorsed several decades earlier by Adelle Davis and Nathan Pritikin (among others), I began to put my patients on a low-fat, high-vitamin diet. "They'll never get their strength back," other doctors told me. "You'll kill them." Ten years earlier, the medical establishment believed that if patients exercised after a heart attack, they would surely die – another assumption now thoroughly discredited.

Some doctors actually threatened to stop referring bypass candidates to me. But by then, I had achieved a solid enough reputation as a surgeon that the patients themselves insisted on seeing me, so my practice didn't suffer. My patients didn't suffer, either. They found that a vegetarian diet did wonders for the heart. They got better faster, and had fewer relapses. They became more vital, they seemed younger – they positively felt *well*.

❖ ❖ ❖ ❖ ❖

Here is the story of how a new treatment for trigeminal neuralgia was born. It is a story of love and science, of life experience and theory. But most important, it is a story of hope for those who suffer with TN and other neurological facial pain.

About the time *The Healing Diet* was published, Janie's sister-in-law Gwen told us about her experience with trigeminal neuralgia, including the lack of helpful treatment she had received so far. Janie and I were both concerned for her, leading us to a new round of clipping, collecting and researching whatever we could find about TN and its current treatments. Over time, we discovered scientific connections between TN and the human body's need for specific nutrients, and Gwen courageously experimented with her diet and supplementation and other holistic regimens we suggested. The results were very encouraging; you can read Gwen's own full account of her experience in Chapter 19.

❖ ❖ ❖ ❖ ❖

Although I have great appreciation for the creativity and diligence of our pharmaceutical industry, it is not surprising that not everything the drug companies tell you is necessarily the whole truth. Medications are not as effective as advertised, and the side effects can be difficult to live with. Occasionally there is a less expensive, safer therapy that can be just as effective as the more radical pharmaceutical or surgical treatments. And even when surgery is required, I have found that natural supplements can help prepare the patient for a surgical intervention. For various reasons – including age, illness, life-style and metabolic individuality – patients can be deficient in one or more micronutrients that could have prevented their diseases in the first place, or that can now help them heal from the ravages of their illnesses.

So it was that through my wife Janie's efforts, my own interest in other medical diseases – and their relationship to nutrition – expanded. She has deepened and broadened how I practice medicine. For years she has been researching information and writing dietary and health-optimizing programs for hundreds of people who asked for her help. When scientific questions arose, she brought me into her deliberations as a resource and consultant. Many of her inquiries and questions were outside my specialty of cardiac surgery, so I had to take a new look at other areas in medicine such as arthritis, cancer, asthma and chronic degenerative diseases.

I reached a startling conclusion as I collated data about these illnesses. The common denominator among all these afflictions is the presence of inflammation and free-radical damage, about which I'll have much more to say throughout this book. The more I worked with these debilitating conditions the more I realized that they can be caused or made more serious – or improved or even cured – by how we eat, think, breathe, work and by the kind of environment we inhabit.

> ❖ ❖ ❖ ❖ ❖
> The common denominator among all these afflictions is the presence of inflammation and free-radical damage

A sense of discovery and excitement is what prompted Janie and me to write this book. Our professional collaboration, however unlikely, has proved very productive.

So if you are suffering with trigeminal neuralgia or other related facial pain, let's get ready to explore some real solutions. The more knowledge you have about these diseases, the better you will understand the process of healing. As a consumer, it is your job to *stay abreast of new information.* I've included several TN patients' brief stories – the stories of people who went from suffering to relief by following the path I've described in this book – which you'll find in Chapter 19. As a consumer it is your job to *be receptive to new opportunities.* Most of this book is devoted to giving you the details of my treatment program—a clear roadmap for how to proceed. As a consumer it is your job to *stay involved in getting well.*

Remember that only you can undertake the journey toward your own good health. You are going to be surprised by how much better you can feel!

PART ONE:

The Trigeminal Neuralgia Puzzle

CHAPTER 1

What Is
Trigeminal Neuralgia?

AN UNCOMMON DISEASE

Trigeminal neuralgia is a severely painful nerve condition that has long defied the medical world's attempts to treat it. It affects the trigeminal nerve, the three-branched system that provides sensation throughout most of the face. TN is an uncommon disease affecting only a small fraction of one percent of all humans – perhaps as few as 50 thousand people among more than 300 million in the United States. It strikes more women than men, mostly after age 60. The failure rate for treatment stands at about 30% – a dismally poor result for modern medicine.

So-called "typical" or "classic" TN is characterized by a severe lightning-like pain that strikes in the eye, cheek or jaw area – or rarely in a combination of these areas. These bolts of pain hit without warning, repeatedly over less than a minute or so, then they stop – only to return and repeat the cycle of misery, often many times per day. This pain is often confused with the symptoms of other ailments such as multiple sclerosis or – very commonly – dental problems. It usually affects only the right side of the face, sometimes only the left side – but very rarely both sides.

It's actually not possible for most people without TN to appreciate the nearly unimaginable intensity of this type of pain. That is one of the most frustrating aspects of having TN – it's so clear that family and friends, while concerned and understanding, really can't fathom how agonizing it is. Suffice to say TN has been described as "the worst pain known to mankind," and as "the suicide disease," since more than a few sufferers have killed themselves to escape the pain.

The causes of this disease are not positively known, but the current hypothesis is that the "typical" TN most often encountered is caused by an artery or vein crossing over and pressing on the trigeminal nerve in the base of the skull and, over time, eroding the nerve's protective covering, or sheath. The resulting "short circuit" in the nerve causes the incredibly painful shocks that shoot through the affected parts of the patient's face. However, in a large percentage of cases, the cause of even this most common type of TN cannot be determined precisely. Erosion of the nerve sheath, called *demyelination*, can often be seen at some distance from where an artery crosses a nerve. Is this the cause? We doctors can't be sure. But we now have strong suspicions that most facial neuralgias share some type of nerve-sheath deterioration as the primary culprit.

Other possible causes of typical TN and atypical facial neuralgias include tumors, cysts, aneurysms, malformed arteries or veins, immature myelin sheath, or a direct injury to a nerve from an accident or a medical procedure. Other medical conditions seem to be associated with facial neuralgias, including multiple sclerosis, Lyme disease, herpes zoster (shingles), chronic degenerative disease (due to aging), infections of the trigeminal ganglion and various nutritional deficiencies. Even more possible causes for myelin destruction include gluten intolerance, a genetic disaffinity for vitamin B12, low levels of melanin and testosterone – or high levels of some toxins, such as lead or mercury.

Clearly, identifying a precise cause for any of these neurological face-pain conditions is a very uncertain business, and routine misdiagnosis is the predictably common result.

Although the *why* of TN and many other types of facial pain remains a puzzle for the medical community, the *how* is remarkably consistent. It is the loss of the protective sheath surrounding the nerve axon brought on by an inflammation which may be initiated by one or more of the possible causes I've just mentioned. In all cases there is evidence of the loss of this nerve-insulating tissue, and of the presence of inflammatory cells in the trigeminal nerve. I will show you a little later why this is such an important phenomenon. But first, let's look at the make-up of the trigeminal nerve.

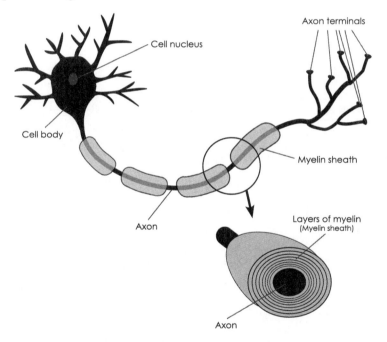

The trigeminal nerve is a bundle of individual nerve fibers twisted on itself in a co-axial fashion. The fibers live in intimate proximity to each other, separated only by their myelin sheath insulation, much as bundled electrical wires are each covered to prevent short-circuits and sparks. The myelin sheath constitutes about 20% to 30% of the weight of these nerve bundles.

Different types of nerve fibers carry different messages. Some send messages to the body causing muscle contractions, for example. Others are sensory, sending messages from the body to the brain so we can recognize sensations such as touch, heat and pain.

When the myelin sheath becomes eroded, bare nerve tissue comes into contact with other bare nerves so that the signal sent to the brain for heat or cold is cross-transmitted to the pain fibers. This causes these non-insulated nerve fibers to send a scrambled message to the brain when stimulated by what should be harmless signals such as a light touch or a mild temperature change. In this case, brushing your teeth, drinking cold water, or feeling a light breeze across your cheek can instantly generate intense pain.

AN OBVIOUS REMEDY

The obvious remedy for this situation is to rebuild the myelin sheath, or at least protect it from further destruction. Once the original insult is eliminated (as after surgery to relieve the effects of a nerve-compressing artery), the body can repair and regenerate the sheath. Nerve tissue has the highest rate of metabolism and nutritional turnover in the body. However, without the proteins, fats, carbohydrates and appropriate enzymes and vitamins necessary for repair, the body cannot adequately regenerate the myelin sheath.

Because there is such a rapid turnover in the nerve fiber and a high metabolic rate, the building blocks, enzymes and catalysts necessary to produce these structures must be readily available for the body either to repair or rebuild damaged nerve tissue. Since these micronutrients and macronutrients work in synergy with each other, it is necessary to have *all* the substances present in order to create the appropriate structures, much in the way one needs cement, sand, and water – in the proper amounts – to make concrete that will not flake or crack. If these various nutrients are not provided in adequate amounts, the tissue repair will be incomplete, or it will occur at a slower pace. Whether the nerve has been de-myelinized due to trauma or erosion, or is defective due to inadequate building material, really does not matter. In either case, *re*-myelination is necessary. The cause of the demyelination is less at issue than the remedy when it comes to relieving the sufferings of the facial neuralgia patient.

> ❖ ❖ ❖ ❖ ❖
> The obvious remedy for this situation is to rebuild the myelin sheath, or else protect it from further destruction.

The appropriate amounts of the various biochemicals, enzymes, vitamins and minerals necessary to properly rebuild nerve tissue depend on the severity of the damage. It also depends on the constitutional makeup of the individual. Today it is well known that repairing nerve damage requires higher levels of micronutrients and macronutrients than nerve maintenance does. There is good evidence that nerve regeneration, including the regulation of protein synthesis, is positively influenced by high doses of vitamin B12, which affect not only the nerve sheath, but the regeneration of the nerve itself.[1]

Sadly, traditional medicine has not yet employed this obvious remedy for facial neuralgias.

---

[1] High school chemistry taught us how a chemical equation is structured. On the left hand side of the equation are two chemicals, and on the right hand side a new compound which is created by the union of these two chemicals. If we add a *catalyst* — a substance that is not used as a part of the new compound, but facilitates the reaction — we can boost the creation of the new compound. The human body does this billions of times each day during the metabolism of its cells. By overloading the availability of all the biologic ingredients, we can greatly increase the amount of the new compound. This reasoning constitutes the bedrock principle of *orthomolecular* medicine, discussed in chapter 14.

CHAPTER 2

A Brief History
Of Treating Facial Pain

WHAT HAS WORKED, AND WHAT HAS NOT

Trigeminal neuralgia, prior to the modern medical era, was known as *tic douloureux,* from the French meaning "a spasm of pain". This describes the severe onset and extreme intensity of this disabling condition. Over the centuries, many remedies were advocated, including venom, arsenic, opiates and hemlock. In the late 19th and early 20th Century, physicians tried radiation, anesthetic inhalation, and injection of many ineffective and sometimes toxic substances.

During this early period of rapid expansion in neurosurgery, surgeons simply cut the entire distribution center of the patient's trigeminal nerve. This brought immediate relief to the patient, but at the cost of various complications such as numbness and dry eye — or in severe cases, even paralysis. Throughout the 1920s and up into the 1960s, many of today's surgical treatments for TN were conceived. Megadoses of injected niacin were first tried in Spain in the 1940s, and by the 1950s, injections of vitamin B12 were first used.

There were also important advances in the pharmaceutical area, with the use of anti-epileptic drugs such as phenytoin (trade name Dilantin) and carbamazepine (Tegretol). More recently, baclofen, Terazol and Neurontin were added to the growing list of drugs being prescribed to control TN and other facial pain.

PROCEDURES

For at least four decades, the "gold standard" surgical treatment for TN has been *microvascular decompression* — MVD for short – a highly invasive procedure.

The principal of microvascular decompression is to correct the problem caused by the slow erosion of the trigeminal nerve's myelin sheath due to the compression of an artery or vein lying across the nerve. The offending blood vessel is lifted off the nerve and a Teflon sheath is placed around the nerve to protect it from further erosion. This requires a complex brain operation which has about ½ % to 1% mortality rate.

Following a microvascular decompression, the chance of being pain free for five years is between 70% and 90%, with about 20% of patients reporting some form of facial pain by the five-year mark. The most common complications after surgery are aseptic meningitis in about 10% of the cases, with hearing loss, headaches, numbness, burning sensation, unsteadiness, dizziness, eye problems and other side effects reported about 25% of the time.[2] Several other operative procedures made at the Gasserian ganglion – the area in front of the ear where the trigeminal nerve splits into its three primary branches — are destructive to the nerve, including balloon compression, glycerol injection or radio frequency lesioning. These have high rates of recurrence and sensory loss including eye complications, double vision, eating problems, motor weakness and *dysesthesia*.[3]

---

[2] If at the time of surgery no vascular compression is found, some surgeons perform a partial sensory rhizotomy, which has a higher rate of failure, higher rate of recurrence and more complications beyond sensory loss.

[3] Peripheral procedures such as interruption or injection with phenol glycerol or other medications have a higher recurrence rate and loss of anesthesia, and are generally less effective in controlling TN pain.

The most recent major "surgical" technique is gamma knife which, under the guidance of magnetic resonance imaging and stereotactic techniques, uses a focused group of cobalt radiation beams to perform a non-invasive incision in the trigeminal nerve. Although recent results are encouraging, it may take up to a year before maximum pain relief is achieved. 17% of gamma knife patients report sensory loss following the procedure, and several studies show a 17% to 34% recurrence rate. Nearly 20% of patients report no benefit at all from their treatment, while the number of pain-free patients two years after treatment ranges from about 60 to 80%. Because this procedure is destructive to the nerve, there is also the risk of other complications including hearing loss and other sensory problems.

> **Def:** *Dysesthesia*: Sensations – heat, cold, tingling – that a patient actually feels, even without the presence of any actual physical stimulation.

MEDICATIONS

Having looked at the risks of all these surgical procedures, I understand why many TN patients choose to take medications to control their pain, even though these powerful drugs have life-changing side effects and a high failure rate. That said, the effects of these medications on the consciousness, awareness and human interaction of TN patients often profoundly impacts their relationships.

> ❖ ❖ ❖ ❖ ❖
>
> Having looked at the risk/benefit ratio of surgical procedures for TN, I understand why many patients opt to take medications to control their pain, even though these powerful drugs have life-changing side effects and a high failure rate

Modern medical therapy for the treatment of trigeminal neuralgia includes these medications, among others (with common brand names capitalized):

Anticonvulsants: phenytoin (Dilantin), carbamazepine (Tegretol), gabapentin (Neurontin), oxcarbazepine (Trileptal) and Lyrica.

Muscle relaxants: baclofen (Lioresal), tizanidine (Zanaflex).

Antidepressants: amitriptyline (Elavil), nortriptyline (Pamelor).

The most common side effects of these medications are dizziness, drowsiness, forgetfulness, unsteadiness and nausea. Rare but serious side effects are also possible: liver toxicity, kidney dysfunction and anemia complications, including flushing, paralysis, recurrence, numbness, dry-eye, and a type of hypersensitivity that is registered in the brain as a kind of 'pins and needles' effect on the skin.

As a whole, the medicinal treatment of trigeminal neuralgia is initially effective in approximately 60% of patients. But this success is often accompanied by intermittent recurrences and by an eventual crossover to the need for surgical intervention for patients exasperated by the side effects of medications, which often are needed in higher and higher doses over time as the underlying condition worsens. All told, only about 25% of TN patients will have long-term relief from medication.

As for surgery, the initial response rate is about 80%, although approximately one-fourth of those patients have some recurrence within one to five years. From the variety of treatments available, none is ideal and there is certainly ample room for improvement.

RESEARCH

Existing treatments for facial pain are well established, with few recent developments in either medicines or procedures. But modern science continues to look for better treatments for facial pain through research, although funds are very limited to support research into any disease that affects relatively few people.

One such research project that shows promise is going on at the University of Florida, where neuroscientist Dr. Lucia Notterpek is engaged in major new studies to address fundamental questions about the role of damage or deterioration of the myelin sheath in trigeminal neuralgia and related facial pain. Her research is funded by the Facial Pain Research Foundation. This is the research arm of TNA/The Facial Pain Association, the world's leading organization in providing patient support, education and research into all types of facial pain.

There is real hope that someday scientists will discover how to control and repair the damage to the nerve's sheath that appears to be at the very center of neuropathic facial pain.

But it is clear to me that for the here and now, if you are suffering from one of these conditions as you read this, if you can control the pain of facial neuralgia with lifestyle changes and supplements, it is preferable in most cases to taking debilitating drugs or undergoing uncertain surgeries.

CHAPTER 3

Your Risk/Benefit Ratio

DOES IT HURT? WILL IT *HARM* ME?
DOES IT HELP? WILL IT *HEAL* ME?

It is common practice in my specialty, cardiothoracic surgery, to evaluate each patient in the light of a "risk/benefit" ratio. As a patient, you should insist that the benefit received from a procedure or medication will far outweigh the risk taken. When we evaluate the risk, we not only look at the possibility of the patient dying, but also the chance of *morbidities,* which are the much more likely complications you might sustain from receiving the treatment. What are the chances of success? What are the chances of recurrence? How much will treatments cost the patient?

These questions help define the impact of any procedure upon the patient's life. A human life must not only be evaluated in terms of longevity. Our lives are not one dimensional. They have breadth of quality as well as length in years. As an example, it would be highly imprudent for a person 20 pounds overweight to undergo gastric stapling because the risks they would take would greatly outweigh any benefit they might receive. Furthermore, the 20-pound weight loss could reasonably be accomplished by a diet and exercise program. On the other hand, a person whose whole life is compromised by morbid obesity might well consider the same procedure when taking into account the risk/benefit ratio.

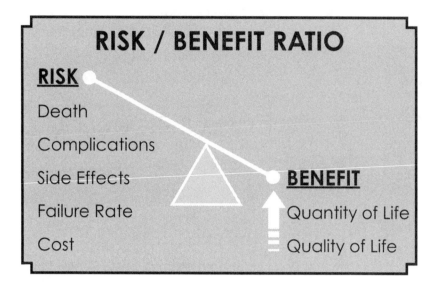

In many diseases, we can almost judge the success or failure of treatment by the number of therapies that are in use. Clearly, TN is a good example of an illness with multiple traditional treatments, most of which present less than optimal outcomes. In reaching for greater success in treatment, greater risk is unavoidable because of the multiple treatments involved and their interactions with one another. This axiom holds true for trigeminal neuralgia: as the success rate of traditional medical treatments increases, so does the magnitude of the risk, the severity of the complications — and even the chance of death.

Recognizing that the most serious complication of death is unlikely, life-shattering events such as stroke, paralysis, facial palsy, pain or recurrent symptoms can all occur, especially during surgical intervention or other high-risk treatments. And there is always the subject of the high cost of these treatments, and whether they are worth that cost.

Even if such major complications do not occur, the side effects of drug therapy may include many debilitating symptoms such as fatigue, drowsiness, nausea, double vision, dizziness, muscle pain, shaking, a "robot-like" or "zombie-like" feeling, and a "fuzzy brain." An estimated 70% of TN patients have side effects from medical therapy. Quite often, these side effects limit the patient's activities, such as preventing safe driving or the ability to function in normal social settings. These side effects can also profoundly affect interpersonal relationships with life partners and family. Some people are allergic to common TN medications and have serious reactions to them. Others can have a mild rash or itching, showing a more mild intolerance to these medications.

ABOUT DRUGS: THE FDA AND "PROOF"

I often hear complaints that the use of integrative and complementary treatments is not "evidence based" and should not be condoned. But as Einstein famously said, "Not everything that can be counted counts, and not everything that counts can be counted." So the lack of evidence of effectiveness is not the same as evidence of lack of effectiveness. Because something is not proven does not mean that it is not true.

It is also interesting that 50% of the medications and equipment that we use daily in standard medical care are not evidence-based and is therefore "off-label" usage, meaning that they have not been approved by the FDA for the therapy for which it is being prescribed.

FDA approval is given after rigorous examination of evidence to verify effectiveness. If a medication is used off-label, it means that there has not been enough evidence submitted to the FDA to support that use, so the use of medications for off-label uses implies that it is not evidence based.

Nearly half of the current clinical practices recommended by the American College of Cardiology and the American

Heart Association are based on expert opinion and on case studies and standards of care which are not evidence based.

A MORE NATURAL APPROACH

Quite often an appointment with a neurologist requires a 4-6 week wait. This period of otherwise lost time could be used as an opportunity to learn whether or not a natural remedy might be successful. There are natural remedies that do not cause complications or raise medical risks for TN patients. Doesn't it make sense to see if undertaking a simple change in diet and micronutrient supplements might prove helpful? Why not attempt to bypass some of the more serious complications that often occur following a more significant intervention? I can't see any downside to this approach.

> ❖ ❖ ❖ ❖ ❖
> There are natural remedies that do not cause complications or raise medical risks for TN patients.

Since we know the complications and side effects of surgical and medical therapy, we should also understand the risks from natural remedies. The good news here is that natural remedies – instead of creating side effects – create side *benefits*. This is because the body responds positively to life-style improvements in diet, exercise and stress modification.

EPIGENETICS

Epigenetics is a new science that has restructured our thinking about genetic involvement and disease. A network of gene locations is involved in changes that create disease. Amazingly, lifestyle changes can actually determine the genetic response, which was previously thought impossible.

The previously accepted idea of a gene malfunction predetermining what illness a person may come down with has been dramatically reassessed. Basically, the principle of epigenetics is that genes respond to the external stimuli of food, toxins, environment, free radicals, stress, exercise and other information, and respond accordingly by suppressing or promoting an increase of enzyme and protein production that dramatically affects the individual's wellness.

An example of this is in cigarette smoking.

EXAMPLE:

Let's look at three heavy cigarette smokers all having a similar human genome with minor variations due to the hereditary contributions from their mothers and fathers.

Patient A: When presented with the information of heavy smoking, the gene pool of patient A translates this information into mutation and Patient A goes on to develop lung cancer through mutation or decreased resistance.

Patient B's gene sees this smoking information and translates it to inflammation of the arterial walls, causing heart disease.

Patient C: The smoking of Patient C is translated to fibrosis and emphysema.

Three patients now have three separate diseases treated by three doctors – an oncologist, a cardiologist and a pulmonologist — with three different forms of therapy. On the surface, their diseases are very separate conditions with strong genetic components. But in taking a closer look, we see that each disease is a genetic response to the impact of smoking.

By removing the smoking we can eliminate the response and therefore eliminate the three diseases.

In terms of risk/benefit, here we see that stopping smoking and other lifestyle changes not only don't have side effects but have side *benefits*—because now a change in diet, exercise or stress modification can affect not only your wellness in the area of heart disease, cancer or emphysema, but can also reduce diabetes, obesity, hypertension, high cholesterol, osteoporosis and arthritis.

PROBLEMS WITH TRADITIONAL TREATMENT

Unfortunately, today doctors are treating symptoms and numbers rather than illness. Obesity, high cholesterol and high blood pressure are not diseases – but they can *lead* to disease, such as stroke or heart attack. These are normal bodily responses to poor life choices. But rather than address causes of the condition, medicine today treats the numbers as if those were actual diseases.

By getting back to a healthy lifestyle, you can change the information that is received by your gene pool and affect positive changes in a variety of chronic degenerative diseases, including heart disease, cancer, arthritis, diabetes, neuropathies and many other illnesses that plague our society today.

Your lifestyle is within your power to control. Of course, there are other situations that adversely affect your health – some of which you may not be able to control — including toxic emissions in our atmosphere and water, depletion of the soil, the amount of hydrocarbons and heavy metals in our environment and many other contaminants.

TREATING SYMPTOMS OR
TREATING CAUSES?

Treating a chronic degenerative disease such as TN with medications, aside from the serious side effects and complications which they may cause, is primarily treating the symptoms and not the cause of the disorder. If the blood pressure is high, we doctors give a pill; if the thyroid is low, we give a pill; if the sugar is high, another pill. This is like cutting the wires to your fire alarm that has just gone off in response to a fire in your basement. Because there is no sound any longer, you assume that the problem has been resolved.

Treating abnormal numbers as if they were diseases does not require a doctor or a nurse — a robot can handle it just as well. I think this is doing a great disservice to our medical community. I believe that because of the way insurance companies are structured today, physicians cannot appropriately serve their patients in the short time they have to care for them. We must seriously re-examine our approach to the wellness of our society.

> ❖ ❖ ❖ ❖ ❖
> Rather than address causes of the condition, medicine today treats the symptoms and numbers as if those were the disease.

Natural remedies approach the *cause* of the disease and attempt to rectify it. Natural complementary or integrative therapies have been shown not only to correct the disease but to offer the additional side benefits of improving other areas of our health.

With all of these side benefits and potential advantages, doesn't it make sense to try an 8 week approach to natural healing of trigeminal neuralgia? From a risk/benefit approach, the answer seems very clear.

Here are a few examples of how natural remedies can not only treat the causes of a medical problem, but can also benefit the body in unexpected ways.

BONUS TERRITORY

Omega 3 oils, found in fish and flax, can decrease the risk of heart disease and heart attacks, improve heart rhythm and help with cholesterol problems. But as side benefits, these same omega 3 oils will also minimize joint aches and pains, improve the musculoskeletal function and decrease inflammation in other organs and body tissues.

Magnesium replacement not only helps control muscle cramps, but improves migraine, asthma, hypertension and many other conditions that are affected by muscle spasm and low magnesium levels.

Vitamin D, which I will talk about at greater length in chapter 15, is beneficial not only to the skeletal system but also to the neurologic, cardiovascular and immune systems.

Exercise, stress modification and proper diet can reduce the risk of cardiovascular disease, cancer, arthritis, osteoporosis, diabetes, hypertension and obesity – and can help moderate all types of facial pain. It can even increase your longevity, and is a strong anti-aging and wrinkle-preventing regimen – real bonus territory!

CHAPTER 4

Inflammation

THE INFLAMMATORY PROCESS

Another basic concept in the nutritional approach to controlling trigeminal neuralgia is the very nature of the inflammatory process itself in the demyelination of the nerve sheath. In not-too-technical detail, local irritation — by trauma, toxins, viruses or bacteria — creates a cascade effect, releasing substances which produce highly reactive and dangerous molecules that in turn destroy the components of the affected cell's membranes and nucleus, and eventually the basic process of the cell itself. The release of these rogue molecules – known as *free radicals* – is known as *oxidative stress*.

The body has many systems for overcoming oxidative stress. It produces its own defensive substances, or it uses ingested vitamins such as A, C and E, as well as mineral catalysts such as selenium, magnesium and zinc. These are commonly known as *antioxidants*. We hear much about antioxidants today related to health and nutrition, even as ingredients in cosmetics and hair products. But most people have no idea what antioxidants actually are, or how important they are to our good health. I'll have much more to say on this subject in chapter 16.

Antioxidants supply a missing electron to "de-fang" a free radical, quenching its role in oxidative stress, and preserving nearby tissue from damage.

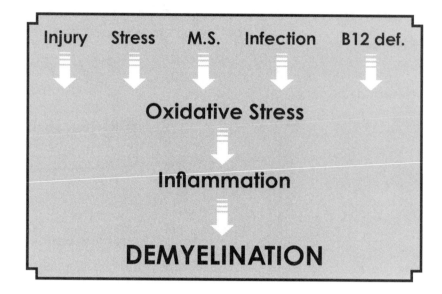

Injury   Stress   M.S.   Infection   B12 def.

Oxidative Stress

Inflammation

DEMYELINATION

OXIDATIVE STRESS – WHAT IS IT?

I can remember going to a carnival as a young boy and watching a fire-eating sword-swallower as he casually belched flames from his mouth without any apparent injury. We were all amazed at this feat and could not figure out how it was done. It was only when I got to medical school that I realized how this stunt works.

In order to burn human tissue, three things are necessary:

1) You must have a flammable substance in an oxygen-rich environment,

2) You need a source of ignition to start a fire,

3) The fire has to be in contact with the tissue long enough to create damage.

This trick works because the fire is quickly doused by the fire-eater before it can do any harm.

Oxidative stress is very much like a fire. In the case of fire, the rapid oxidation (electron transfer) of a burning substance produces energy in the form of light and heat. Oxidative stress in the body, although a slower process, also involves the exchange of electrons. This forms a new oxidized substance, and energy is released, usually in the form of heat. If you limit the amount of oxidizing toxins, or decrease the time the tissue is exposed to them, you will minimize or prevent the inflammatory process.

The oxidizing substance that most commonly tries to steal an electron from our vital tissues is called a *free radical*. These free radicals can result from ingested toxins (created by an interaction of the tissue with a substance such as radiation, heat, or light), or they can be produced by the body itself. This process is not necessarily bad; in fact, the way our white blood cells kill bacteria that invade our body is by this very same process, since the production of free radicals destroys the offending organism. In other words, the production of free radicals in our bodies leads to the destruction of the disease. Free radicals also are produced as a by-product of the natural metabolic process of a cell. Consider this: about 3% of the energy released in the metabolism of the cell is converted to free-radical production.

Oxidative stress is another matter. You can readily see an example of oxidative stress if you cut an apple in half and leave it on the table for a few minutes. You will notice the smooth, white flesh of the apple turning brown. This is the chemical transformation of the apple's cut surface into an oxidized form. The free radicals in the air (oxygen) are in constant search of electrons. When they come into contact with the apple's tissue, they steal electrons from molecules in the cell membrane. Or, if they invade the cell, they steal a molecule from inside the nucleus. When this happens, that molecule takes an electron from the molecule next to it and a chain reaction begins, destroying a large portion of the membrane and proteins in the cell. This allows an influx of toxic substances, which prevents the cell from producing much-needed products.

The inflammation that occurs in this escalating battle is the result of the body producing powerful substances to wall off the area under attack in an attempt to create a positive environment so that the body may limit the damage. Chronic inflammation and long exposure to these substances cause the death of the cells in the involved tissue. Thus, chronic inflammation has been implicated not only in heart disease, but in cancer, arthritis, autoimmune disease and neurologic disorders including trigeminal neuralgia.

> ❖ ❖ ❖ ❖ ❖
> Chronic inflammation has been implicated not only In heart disease, but in cancer, arthritis, autoimmune disease and neurologic disorders, including trigeminal neuralgia.

Fortunately, nature's way of counteracting these electron-scavenging free radicals is to provide them with molecules that can offer up an electron and thus prevent damage to our body's tissues. These molecules are generated within our body from enzyme systems. We call these very helpful molecules *antioxidants.*

Most antioxidants, including a host of plant-derived nutrients and vitamins A, C and E — and several minerals including magnesium and zinc – enter our bodies in the foods we eat. Antioxidants such as co-enzyme Q10 – an important molecule I'll talk more about later – and serum proteins like albumin are produced within our bodies. These substances all can donate electrons to free radicals and quench their need, preserving the integrity of our body tissue.

VITAMIN SYNERGY

Vitamins work in synergy with each other to fight free-radical damage, as in the case of vitamin C. Vitamin C requires vitamin E to acquire an electron from it in the place of the one it has lost. Vitamin E in turn depends on other substances to offer it an electron. This is why many studies which test for the effectiveness of a single antioxidant are not successful. Antioxidants cannot be effective in a vacuum. It is vital to have our tissue primed with vitamins, minerals and enzyme systems in order to counteract the oxidative stress that bombards each cell an estimated 10,000 times a day. Heavily publicized studies have failed to prove or disprove the efficacy of certain vitamins (most recently vitamin E), because they focus on the benefit of the *isolated* vitamin.

> ❖ ❖ ❖ ❖ ❖
> It is vital to have our tissue primed with vitamins, minerals and enzymes to counteract the oxidative stress that bombards each cell 10,000 times a day.

Setting up these studies in order to prove the benefits of an isolated integer unit in a system is a little like telling Tiger Woods, "Tiger, the most important club in your bag is the putter. You're scheduled for a match with Ernie Els today. Now go out there, using only your putter, and prove it!" Obviously, it is *all* the clubs working together, in synergy, supporting each other, that bring about victory in golf. So it is that a variety of antioxidants are needed in order to supply, create, store and donate electrons in the liquid, solid, water or oil phases of our body.

Vitamins are enzymatic protein compounds essential to life that we cannot produce in our bodies. They must be ingested to serve as coenzymes and catalysts in the millions of processes that are required incessantly to create, repair and nourish the billions of cells that constitute our bodies.

Of course, it's best when we can get these vitamins naturally from our food supply, for several important reasons:

First, they work best together — as they are integrated in nature.

Second, scientists don't yet know all the antioxidants and facilitators present in our food, so ingesting them in their natural state gives us the best chance for these vitamins to work at their maximum efficiency.

Third, manufactured or extracted vitamins may not be as beneficial as those from natural sources. They may contain contaminants or inaccurate amounts, and they may lack necessary facilitators to work their best.

Fourth, large doses of some vitamins may be harmful.

Lastly, some vitamins can interfere with certain drugs, and vice versa. 500 of the most-prescribed drugs will have a negative effect on vitamin efficacy. Conversely, more than half of these drugs can themselves be affected by vitamins.

Vitamins greatly facilitate the biologic processes in our body and must be ingested on a regular basis in order to prevent disease conditions such as scurvy, berri-berri, pellagra and a host of other illnesses. These nutritional diseases are the end result of long-standing depravation of specific vitamins.

There are other disease states and chronic conditions that can be initiated or aggravated by a chronic insufficiency of some of these vitamins. Some examples of this are fetal spina bifida in folic-acid-deficient mothers, thrombophlebitis in B-vitamin-deficient patients, and increased arthritic symptoms in omega 3 deficiency. Furthermore, medication may inordinately deplete some micronutrients from our system such as B-vitamin depletion in women who are taking birth control pills, loss of magnesium in patients taking diuretics, co-enzyme Q10 loss deficiency in patients on statin drugs, and vitamin B12, calcium and vitamin D deficiency in patients taking Metformin or H2 blockers.

In order to rebuild healthy tissue, a higher dose of any specific micronutrient is required than the usual maintenance dose, or the dose suggested that prevents the classical symptoms of end-stage diseases, such as scurvy.

CHAPTER 5

Toxins and Stress

TOXINS

When I discuss toxic substances, I am talking about those which are ingested, inhaled or made contact with through any series of events that causes degenerative disease. These toxic agents can affect the nervous system as well as many other bodily functions. Since the nervous system contains a significant amount of lipid molecules, substances such as organic hydrocarbons are most toxic to the nerve tissue because they are not only readily absorbed by the nerves but – once there – are difficult to remove.

Toxic substances can be ingested or produced within the body whenever the metabolism is in a deficiency state. This is a vital concept to underscore as we look for the cures to chronic degenerative disease. These diseases, including trigeminal neuralgia, can only develop if an initiating factor intrudes from the outside of the body, or if a toxic substance is produced from within. Toxins which come from the outside environment include gases such as carbon monoxide, heavy metals such as mercury, or liquids such as alcohol. Inside toxicity occurs from certain neurotransmitters

❖ ❖ ❖ ❖ ❖

Toxic substances can harm the body in three ways:

1) When ingested, they can directly damage cells.

2) When they build up within the body, the body's metabolism can produce a harmful reaction as it attempts to clear them out.

3) They can react within the cells, where the cells can produce a harmful byproduct in reaction to contact with the toxins.

like glutamate, which at high levels will cause toxicity and cell death. Indeed, some neurotoxins like botulism have been used to block the trigeminal nerve, and other attempts at nerve destruction use chemicals like glycerol to try to eliminate pain.

For optimum nerve health in the treatment of trigeminal neuralgia, it is important to minimize your exposure to certain environmental and ingested toxic substances. Generally, these toxic substances fall into three categories: organic hydrocarbons, heavy metals and *excitotoxins*, about which I'll have more to say shortly.

The reason exposure to these toxins should be minimized is that all of them will cause increased excitability and derangement of normal metabolism in the nervous system. This can cause the fragile equilibrium of the temporarily pain-free trigeminal neuralgia patient to be broken by an increase in free radicals created by the toxins, setting off a fresh outbreak of TN pain.

We are constantly bombarded with organic hydrocarbons from industrial byproducts, fuel combustion, organic solvents and chlorinated amino acids. These products are found very commonly in our drinking water, in our soil – even in the air we breathe. Billions of pounds of byproducts from the burning of gasoline, heating oil, diesel fuel and coal are spewed into the atmosphere each year. The chloride in our water sources interacts with the organic material in our reservoirs to form harmful chloro-organic chemicals. Harmful compounds such as bisphenol-A, used in making plastic beverage bottles, can leach into the liquids inside – and end up in our bodies. All of these toxins increase oxidative stress and free-radical formation, which cause inflammation in our bodies and can lead to a worsening of trigeminal neuralgia symptoms.

The same is true for heavy metals, especially mercury and lead. Lead is also a neurotoxic substance once used in making paint and gasoline; its serious effects on humans have long been well known.[4]

Chlorine is another highly toxic element that causes oxidative stress when introduced into the body. Organic chlorides are even worse, and many *perchlorates,* which are created as byproducts of food production, can inhibit thyroid function.

Inhaled toxins such as smoke, smog and petrochemicals can cause tremendous oxidative stress of the tissue within the lungs, which then creates inflammatory reactions leading to the breakdown of adjacent areas. Insecticides can be neurotoxic and, with the great influx of foreign-produced foods, we must be extremely careful about product contamination with insecticides that are not approved for use in our country.

❖ ❖ ❖ ❖ ❖
All of these substances increase oxidative stress and free radical formation, which cause inflammation in our body and can exacerbate trigeminal neuralgia.

Even locally grown foods may have taken up more lead from their soil than foods grown far away, following decades of contamination from the residue of lead paint and ethyl gasoline. So it pays to be ever-vigilant about all of our food – reading labels very carefully and certainly minimizing the amounts of processed foods that we eat.

Mercury is concentrated in fish – especially older, larger fish which have ingested it from the spillage of chemicals in our rivers and oceans. Fifty percent of all mercury in the environment comes from the burning of coal, which drives the vaporized mercury into the atmosphere, there to combine with rain, and be washed into the rivers and oceans. This is the largest

---

[4] Lead or mercury poisoning is often treated by a process called *chelation* in which an agent known as EDTA is used to clear the heavy metals from the tissues.

source of mercury contamination in the world. I believe it is wise to avoid eating swordfish steaks, large tuna and shark meat, as these predators may have lived as long as twenty years in polluted waters, concentrating the mercury collected in the small fish they eat.

Since no animal can properly excrete the mercury it ingests, any other animal that eats these creatures will also be ingesting their mercury intake, and so on up the food chain. My advice is: when choosing fish, stick to younger salmon, trout or other small fish.

I would also recommend reading food labels very carefully for another reason: avoiding high-fructose corn syrup. Why? In January, 2009, the Institute for Agriculture and Trade Policy found that nearly 50% of the tested samples of commercial high-fructose corn syrup contained mercury. Another study found detectible levels of mercury in 45% of commercial high-fructose corn syrup samples.

A separate study detected mercury in one-third of 55 popular brand-named products where high-fructose corn syrup is the first or second ingredient by volume – cola drinks, candies, jams and the like – including products by Coke, Quaker, Hershey, Kraft and J.M. Smucker.

In recent years, high-fructose corn syrup has increasingly replaced sugar as a sweetener even in many processed foods where sweeteners are not a primary ingredient, including snacks, breads, cereals, lunch meats, yogurts, soups and condiments. On average, an American consumes about twelve teaspoons per day – even higher amounts for teenagers, up to 80% more than the average.

Some more bad news about high-fructose corn syrup is that caustic soda is used in scrubbing the corn starch from the corn kernel, using a product which contains chlorine and aluminum. There are traces of these elements in much of the high-fructose corn syrup used today. So we all must be extremely cautious about all the processed foods we eat and drink.

EXCITOTOXINS

Excitotoxins are a newly identified source of oxidative stress for nerve tissue. The "Chinese food syndrome" described some 40 years ago was attributed to the use in cooking of monosodium glutamate – MSG. The offending agent in this compound is glutamate, which "excites" the nerve cells and causes hyper-irritability, excitability and eventually nerve death. O t h e r neurotoxins have now been identified, including certain amino acids, partially hydrogenated amino acids, and aspartame, a sugar substitute. Diet sodas and diet foods should be sparingly consumed, since they do often contain this potentially toxic substance. Aspartame has been linked not only to neurotoxicity, but may also even be carcinogenic.

So it is absolutely essential for us to be very cautious about the toxins that are found both in our environment and in the foods we eat. If we can reduce the excitability of our nerves and reduce inflammation and free-radical formation that tends to worsen the demyelination process in trigeminal neuralgia, we will have taken some important steps toward healing.

CHAPTER 6

Lymphatics and
The Immune System

THE LYMPHATIC SYSTEM

The lymphatic system is closely involved in preventing or reducing the inflammatory process, regardless of its origin.

If the primary cause of inflammation is bacterial or viral in origin, the lymphatics are necessary to recruit appropriate cells and antibodies to destroy the viruses and bacteria.

The most important of the immune process delivery systems, the lymphatics must be continually detoxified if the entire immune system is to function correctly.

> ❖ ❖ ❖ ❖ ❖
> During oxidative stress, it is important for the lymphatics to remove cellular debris from intercellular spaces.

Good lymphatic flow is also essential for the transmission of messenger systems from the affected tissue to the lymph nodes and thymus, which produce bacteria- and virus-resisting cells and substances – a kind of bodily early-warning system.

In case of high cholesterol levels, the lymph is vital in both circulating and increasing the amount of "good" HDL to which the "bad" cholesterol can then be exposed and eventually eliminated from the body.

In times of oxidative stress, it is important for the lymphatics to remove cellular debris from intercellular spaces so that the amount of time the debris is in contact with the tissue of the organ is limited and the peroxides and free radicals are cleared from the tissue.

THE IMMUNE SYSTEM

To understand the effects of toxins, we have to know how the immune system works. Immunity can be either *specific* or *non-specific*. Nonspecific immunity is the body's reaction to any outside substance not derived from within the body itself. The body can recognize a foreign protein or organism that has entered, and it has the innate ability to attack and destroy that toxic substance. Specific immunity derives from our body's "memory" of having been introduced to the same outside toxic substance in the past. The body stores in its cells and fluids ways to react against that specific outside invader, and when it encounters the substance again, it attacks.

The two types of specific immunity are called *cell-mediated* and *humoral* immunity. Cell-mediated immunity is the process by which the cells directly engage with the outside substances, attacking and destroying them. In humoral immunity, our body recognizes the foreign substance and then creates antibodies to circulate in the body fluids, which will attach to any invading substance and destroy it. This ability is based on the recognition by the body of the foreign substance – its "memory."

Cells that create antibodies are called *plasma cells*. Plasma cells live in the lymphatic system and lymph nodes. They identify foreign substances and then manufacture Y-shaped proteins called *antibodies* that will lock onto the foreign invaders and destroy them. These antibodies float freely in the blood and lymphatic systems and are also attached to the membranes of plasma cells, so that when they come into contact with toxic substances they can lock the plasma cells onto them.

ANTIBODIES

Five main classes of antibodies can be distinguished, each with a different purpose:

1. *Immunoglobulin G (IgG)* antibodies pursue foreign proteins called antigens and are the most common type found in the body. They are produced late in the immune response, so that when they're seen, it's a sign of an established infection.

2. *Immunoglobulin M (IgM)* antibodies signal recent infection. They are initially mobilized when bacteria or viruses invade the body.

3. *Immunoglobulin E (IgE)* antibodies come into play in allergic reactions such as asthma, eczema, and hay fever.

4. *Immunoglobulin A (IgA)* antibodies are found in saliva, tears, and the mucous membranes of the gastrointestinal tract. They are a defense against proteins and bacteria invading the mucosa or the bowels.

5. *Immunoglobulin D (IgD)* is a little-known antigen that has arcane functions. It is still under investigation, but researchers are optimistic about its beneficial effects.

COMMUNICATION

The immune system communicates through *peptides* – partial proteins made of *amino acids*, which are the precursors of protiens – and proteins, secreted by one cell and received by another. These messenger chemicals proceed along the body's systemic pathways.

The messenger substances include *cytokines* (meaning "cell movement"), proteins that take about four to six hours for the body to manufacture, and *polypeptides* or *neuropeptides*, both consisting of amino acids. The peptides take less time to manufacture and thus are more quickly available for the immune system to use.[5]

The most amazing thing is that nerve cells, immune cells, and endocrine cells all have receptors not only for their own messages, but also for those of other systems. The nervous system, for example, has receptors for both the immune and the endocrine messages that are coming in. That's how information is exchanged at the cellular level, and how your immune system can affect your neurological system and vice-versa. In this way, TN can cause an episode of depression, and depression can cause a TN flare-up.

❖ ❖ ❖ ❖ ❖
TN can cause an episode of depression, and depression can cause a TN flare-up.

THE IMMUNOLOGIC PROCESS

This is how the body goes into all-out defensive warfare – just wade though this medical lingo to get a feel for the breathtaking cellular activity involved:

Assume that a virus or some form of bacterium has gained access to your body, where it has started growing and multiplying. A macrophage engulfs it, processes the proteins on its membranes, and then takes the antigen – which has made the organism unique – and passes it to a helper T cell, which binds it to the macrophage. This union causes the macrophage to release messenger proteins that work to activate quiescent T cells. From

---

[5] **The Body's Messengers:**
   Endocrine messengers are substances released for a general purpose in a far-off area.
   Exocrine messengers are secreted in a tube or "duct" (and into the bile duct).
   Paracrine messengers are local molecules that regulate between two cells in a local area, or they stimulate other immune activity.
   Each messenger system is specific as to which cell membrane it fits – it's called the "key and lock" theory. Part of a messenger fits into the cell's "lock," like a docking lock on a spacecraft, and turns the "key." The cell membrane then opens or activates another program or secretes something into the system.

them, B cells are stimulated to participate in the response. The B cells will continue secreting antibodies and humoral factors until they are told by suppressor cells that they are no longer needed; then the immune system returns to normal, the invader having been vanquished.

The lymphatics play a vital role in this process. Remember, unless secreted directly into the bloodstream, all the messenger proteins and the intermediary metabolites and toxic waste created by this interaction must be processed through the lymphatics and on into the liver or kidneys. Indeed, many of the immune cells and messenger-producing cells reside in the lymphatic system, and the lymphatic system must be able to get these messengers and immune cells to various parts of the immune system.

> ❖ ❖ ❖ ❖ ❖
> If the lymphatic system is slowed down, the initial reaction to the invading organism is severely impaired.

If the lymphatic system is slowed down, the initial reaction to the invading organism is severely impaired. The "call to alarm" cannot be circulated to the cells, so their response is delayed or diminished, and the toxins – produced by the interaction of the body with the invading protein – stay in the tissue, creating a more hyperactive response from the tissue. This in turn causes greater tissue damage, which delays the message for the suppressor T cells to deregulate their activity, creating a prolonged overreaction in the tissue. In fact, an autoimmune process can then follow, by which the protein of your *own* body is partially broken down, no longer recognized by the immune cells, and then processed as a foreign protein, beginning a long process of inflammatory reaction and "auto-destruction" of your healthy tissues and cells.

THE IMMUNE RESPONSE

The linchpins of nonspecific immunity are the *phagocytes*, white cells that ingest other cells or microorganisms, debris, and proteins from old and dead cells. Phagocytes and other related cells are deeply involved in any general immune response. They are aided by the nonspecific cytotoxic cells – "natural killer cells" – which destroy malignant or bacterial cells by direct contact.

Complement proteins circulate in the bloodstream and also enhance the immune response. Once they are triggered by a foreign substance or organism, their enzymes digest the edges of the foreign protein and attract white cells to the area of inflammation. The complement cascade can be activated by more than just bacteria. In heart-lung surgery, for example, the rough surfaces of the plastic tubes in the heart-lung machine can create a series of reactions by the white cells and complement proteins that cause a total body inflammatory reaction, which can lead to adult respiratory distress syndrome (ARDS), stroke, and renal and/or liver failure. What is normally good for the body sometimes can also become harmful.

> ❖ ❖ ❖ ❖ ❖
> What is normally good for the body sometimes can also become harmful.

LYMPHATICS AS STOREHOUSES

Over and over again during the immune system's response, we see the importance of the lymphatics. Besides being a waste-removal system for all the body's tissues, they also serve as storehouses for immune cells and substances that destroy invading organisms, thus acting to isolate and neutralize toxins. The lymph nodes filter particulate matter, like bacteria and carbon particles, removing them from circulation. In this way, the lymphatic system serves not only as a clearinghouse and filter system, but also as an emergency switchboard where the signal of a messenger substance or alarm from some area of the tissue will mobilize the lymphocytes and the cytokines to react to harmful substances circulating in the body.

DETOXIFICATION

Each of us has a maximum level of tolerance to toxicity that cannot be exceeded if we expect to maintain good health. We've seen how the immune process works to eliminate toxins. This chapter has focused on the care and maintenance of the most important part of the immune-process delivery systems – the lymphatics – which must be continually detoxified if the entire immune system is to function correctly.

> ✧ ✧ ✧ ✧ ✧
> We can reduce the tissue-damaging free radicals that may lead to sometimes fatal inflammation

Stagnant or inadequate lymph flow can impair the immune process, as we've seen, but this weakness is also associated directly with the onset of many symptoms and illnesses including arthritis, bursitis, joint stiffness, dry or flaking skin, lethargy, depression and other more serious diseases including cancer.

I'll be discussing antioxidants in detail in chapter 16, but it's important now to recognize that nature provides us with antioxidants for every potential situation in which oxidative stress may occur. For example, in the lipoprotein that carries cholesterol, a large amount of vitamin E and *ubiquinone* (also known as coenzyme Q10, or just CoQ10) is present to prevent oxidation in the lipids while they are being transported to the tissue. But sometimes these protective amounts are not enough. If we can keep our antioxidant level well elevated in the tissues through good diet, stress reduction, exercise, and supplemental vitamin intake, we can reduce the effects of tissue-damaging free radicals that may lead to sometimes fatal inflammation, and control the bad effects of oxidized cholesterol.

IT'S ABOUT PERSONAL CHOICE

The average American is *choosing* to follow an unhealthy diet filled with processed food, trans-fats, sugar, salt, cheese and refined grains. We consume more soft drinks (more than 600 bottles per person each year) than water. On average, we eat 150 pounds of sugar and 37 pounds of cheese per person per year.

In spite of what we know of the many benefits of fruits and vegetables, only 30% of the population eats five portions per day, and less than one person in ten eats the recommended seven to nine portions a day. And as for the "Top Ten" calorie providers in the average American diet, they are *all* processed foods.

Top Ten Sources of Calories in the American Diet

1. Whole milk
2. Cola (corn syrup)
3. Margarine
4. White bread
5. Rolls, ready to serve
6. Sugar
7. Milk (2% milk fat)
8. Ground beef
9. Wheat flour (white)
10. Pasteurized processed American cheese

Add to that poor diet a lack of exercise and poor stress management and you have a "perfect storm" of bodily conditions that are more likely to increase our free radicals and promote oxidative stress, causing damaging inflammation. Individual and varying genetic response to that inflammation can lead to cell mutation and cancer, arterial inflammation and heart disease, insulin resistance or degeneration of the myelin sheath.

In managing the symptoms of your trigeminal neuralgia or related facial pain, I can hardly over-emphasize the importance of improving your lifestyle in these three critical areas of diet, stress management and exercise – the details of which are the subjects of the next several chapters I firmly believe that not only can you control your neuralgia symptoms, but you can actually reverse the course of the disease itself over time. Be patient, be diligent with improving your lifestyle, take a positive attitude – and watch how much more you will enjoy life!

> ❖ ❖ ❖ ❖ ❖
> I firmly believe that not only can you control your neuralgia symptoms, but you can actually reverse the course of the disease itself over time.

PART TWO:

The Lemole Recovery Program
For Trigeminal Neuralgia

CHAPTER 7

Important Food Facts

SOME BASICS ABOUT DIET

If you had a brand new Rolls-Royce and filled its gas tank every week with kerosene, people would think you were crazy. But everyday those same people fill the most exquisite machine ever devised, the human body, with junk foods and toxins. Our food intake has been so skewed by personal preference ("I'll eat it because it tastes good") and so depleted by processing and the exhausting of micronutrients that our bodies are being swamped with toxins and empty calories while being denied the building blocks for making the enzymes that could nullify oxidative stress and retard aging.

This chapter is about the building blocks that are needed for good health, and particularly about nutrition as it applies to trigeminal neuralgia.

The diet for the trigeminal neuralgia patient varies somewhat from the optimum health diet in that the patient requires a larger amount of "good" fats on the menu in order to build up the myelin sheath that is under repair. It requires more of the fundamental building blocks to repair the nerve sheath than to maintain it under usual circumstances, so it is important to have a higher amount of useful fats in your diet.

I have seen TN patients who were pain free for long periods of time and went on a low fat diet only to have a recurrence of their symptoms. When put on a modified diet with more fats, their symptoms abated. Nevertheless, the objective is still to have a largely plant-based diet with more vegetable oils and fish oils, and fewer meats and dairy products. Adding young cold-water fish such as wild salmon or mackerel can benefit the reparative process.

I recommend not eating conventionally farmed fish because they are deprived of the Omega 3 fatty acids that wild fish have in their diets, and are often pumped with antibiotics and toxic hydrocarbons. Cold-water fish must have Omega 3 oils to keep their temperature constant and to be more flexible in icy waters. They receive these oils from eating plankton, small algae and other sea life. The farmed fish are raised in man-made environments and are fed corn and meal high in Omega 6 oils, which are pro-inflammatory. Because of this, their immune system is diminished and they need antibiotics to survive to adulthood. Many farmed salmon have their flesh artificially colored to look more "natural" because they don't get the natural nutrients that produce the vibrant colors in wild salmon. In general, it makes good sense to avoid conventionally farm-raised fish.[6]

> ❖ ❖ ❖ ❖ ❖
>
> The objective is to have largely a plant-based diet with more vegetable oils and fish oils and fewer meats and dairy products.

Generous portions of avocado, nuts and many other plants are beneficial to the TN patient. Coconut oil is particularly intriguing, as it is good for cooking and contains a saturated fat that is not harmful as are those fats found in meats and dairy products.

---

[6] Great strides are being made in fish farming in several North Atlantic countries, including Norway, Sweden and Scotland. Here, salmon are being cold-water farmed in ocean pens along the seacoasts, where they feed at least partly on naturally available food that moves freely from the seas into the penned areas where these fish are contained. Some growers use no supplemental feeds, and so they are certified organic farmers.

These farmed fish are often highest in Omega 3 fats of all salmon, even higher than many wild varieties. Look for them at specialty purveyors and even some mainline grocers; they are a real treat!

It is important to look at the "color wheel" of fruits and vegetables. The greater range of colors gives us greater amounts of *phytonutrients* for our bodies. Phytonutrients are those chemicals that plants have created over long periods of time to protect themselves from viruses, bacteria, funguses and mutation. These phytochemicals are found in the pigment of the vegetable or fruit, thus the different colors. The more pigmented foods we eat, the more phytonutrients we ingest and may derive the same benefits that the plant does.

Processed foods cannot match these benefits since the phytonutrients are destroyed or neutralized during food processing, rendering such components as fiber, vitamins and enzymes either diminished or destroyed.

EAT A RAINBOW

The colors of vegetables and fruits often provide clues to identifying the unique nutrient or compound that is found in any given plant. Here are some examples of fruits and vegetables that make up the Eating Rainbow.

Dark Green Vegetables – infused with antioxidants, and contain vitamins A, C, and K, folate, iron, calcium, and fiber.

Dark Leafy Greens – Okra – Chard – Watercress

Avocado – Broccoli – Spinach – Romaine Lettuce – Kiwifruit

Artichoke – Arugula – Asparagus – Green Beans – Kale

Red Vegetables And Fruit – contain Lycopene.

Beets – Kidney Beans – Tomatoes – Cherries – Red Peppers

Raspberries – Strawberries – Red Cabbage – Cranberries

Blue And Dark Purple Plants – contain anticancer pigment anthocyanin, as well as antioxidants, fiber, flavanoids and vitamin C.

Blueberries – Blackberries – Elderberries – Purple Figs

Plums – Grapes – Rhubarb – Purple Grapes – Black Beans

Orange And Yellow Plants – contain calcium and promote healthy joints, bones, and eyes.

Sweet Potatoes – Oranges – Squash & Pumpkin – Cantaloupe

Apricots – Carrots – Peaches – Yellow Squash – Corn

White – some contain phytochemicals such as allicin (onions), glucosinolates (cauliflower) and flavanoids.

Onions – Parsnips – Mushrooms – Cabbage – Brussels Sprouts

Cauliflower – Bananas – Garlic – Potatoes – Ginger

Some Important Nutrients Found In Fruit And Vegetables

- ❖ *Beta carotene* is converted in the body to vitamin A. Beta carotene has been associated with promoting healthy eyesight, but has also been associated with cholesterol and triglyceride control.

- ❖ *Lycopene* is found primarily in tomatoes and has been associated with a decreased risk in prostate cancer and heart disease. Lycopene is more readily absorbed when cooked , so lycopene absorption is greater from, say, spaghetti sauce than it is from raw tomatoes.

- ❖ *Lutein* is found in blueberries and squash, and is important for eye health and – along with its relative phytonutrient, _zeaxyxanthin_ – is used to control the development of macular degeneration and cataracts.

❖ *Vitamin C* is a very powerful antioxidant found in vegetables and fruits –especially citrus fruits. It is important in reducing inflammation, quenching free-radical formation, promoting collagen integrity, joint and muscle strength and wound healing.

❖ *Potassium*, a mineral found in great quantities in vegetables, is important for our general well being. The body requires a great amount of potassium to prevent heart disease and hypertension and balance the pH of our blood. However, today's processed-food diets substitute sodium for potassium to preserve foods and create longer shelf-life. Most of the processed foods we eat are depleted of potassium.

❖ *Quercitin*, found in citrus fruits, apples and onions is important for cholesterol metabolism and is also an antioxidant useful for patients with asthma or other breathing problems.

❖ *Bioflavanoids* are found in fruits such as lemons, oranges and limes, which also have high amounts of vitamin C.

❖ *Anthocyanins* are found in fruits and vegetables with a blue or red hue. These compounds are flavanoids important in maintaining nervous-tissue integrity. Blackberries and strawberries are excellent sources of anthocyanins. It would be beneficial in maintaining nerve health – a critical issue to TN patients – to eat a lot of berries. Anthocyanins are powerful antioxidants found to slow the growth of tumor cells.

❖ *Fiber* is found in essentially all plants. We only ingest about 5 grams of fiber a day in the average American diet, but we need at least 30 to 40 grams a day. This can be found in grains, in fruits and vegetables and in the pectin of citrus fruits. Fiber clears us of our excess cholesterol, reduces the risk of GI cancers and helps prevent heart disease. The processed foods we eat today are almost devoid of fiber, although it is often said that meat is high in fiber due to its connective tissue. This couldn't be further from the truth. *Ligins* are the polyphenol components of seeds, flax and other similar food sources. They are beneficial in preventing and controlling cancer and in creating overall hormonal balance.

In considering nutrition and TN, I believe that it is necessary to present the body with all the building blocks needed for the repair and maintenance of the nerve's myelen sheath – the fatty acids, minerals, vitamins and proteins. I believe it is also very helpful to maintain good general nutrition as you focus on healing. This gives your body the best possible chance to regain your good health.

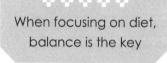

When focusing on diet, balance is the key

THE DIET FOR OPTIMUM HEALTH

When I advocate a diet program to promote health, fight degenerative disease, and generally lead to physical and spiritual well-being, I approach it in several ways.

The first way is to return our lives to a holistic state of balance. The objective should be to support ourselves in all areas of our life rather than focus on diet alone. But even when focusing on diet, balance is the key. It's why I'm so against fad diets, eating the same foods at every meal, or fasting. Yes, I have advocated eating little or no meat, dairy products, cheese, or cake, but there remains a vast array of foods that will guarantee variety and enjoyment.

We should take the time to savor our meals, to be aware of the taste and texture of what we eat, the benefits each mouthful gives us, and the wonderful blessings we get from eating. It's important to integrate our spiritual, mental, and physical environment by being cognizant of the time and love that went into the preparation of our food, and by relaxing during the meal so that it is not tainted by negative emotions like anger or anxiety. Also, we should take our time. When we gulp down our meals, we deny ourselves pleasure, and what good is life without pleasure?

Second, we should decrease or eliminate the toxins in our foods. For most people, a healthy diet would consist of high-complex-carbohydrate meal with about 20 percent fat and 15 percent protein. People suffering from TN should have somewhat more fats, perhaps 25%, but these should be the good fats – the omega 3's and healthy omega 6's. Until recently, however, the Standard American Diet – SAD (how true!) – was about 50 percent fat, 20 percent protein, and 30 percent mostly simple carbohydrates. As noted, the low-fat fads of recent years have changed the percentages, but it has meant that our sugar consumption has grown to about 150 pounds per person each year. Substitution of artificial sweeteners is no solution. They can be carcinogenic and neurologically damaging.

And isn't salt a toxin? It is, and salt in the SAD is up to almost 9 grams a day, most of it hidden in the processed foods and drinks we Americans consume on a daily basis. Salt can cause hypertension and its attendant problems. Sugar has been linked to cancer, heart disease, and a variety of infections. It has been shown to elevate the triglycerides, lower HDL, decrease the white cell immune response, and generally cause great

✧ ✧ ✧ ✧ ✧
MACRONUTRIENTS –
the building blocks –
carbohydrates, fats
and protein

bodily harm. The simplest way to avoid these toxins is to read package labels and avoid foods high in fat, sugar, or salt. Another way is to follow the diet proposed in this book.

Third, I recommend certain rules of thumb in deciding what foods to choose. These are only general guidelines which certainly don't apply to 100 percent of the population, but they are a good starting point.

1) *Use absence of color as an indicator of low nutritional worth.* Avoid white foods—sugar, bleached white flour products (white bread, bagels and pasta), milk, ice cream, cheese, and other milk products. These are processed foods and high-fat, high-cholesterol dairy products. We should keep processed foods in our diet to a minimum because they contain only empty calories from simple carbohydrates, which is all that's left once the vitamins and minerals have been processed away. If you must eat yogurt, milk, ice cream, or cheese, switch to low-fat or fat-free varieties. While it's important to get enough calcium to avoid osteoporosis, be aware that the fat and protein in dairy products can actually leach calcium out of the body. It's far better to use calcium supplements and to substitute soy milk or rice milk for cow's milk. Casein is one of the "best" foods to induce cancer in laboratory animals.

2) *Three times a week, eat a dinner limited to plants only.* Eating more vegetables and fruits can reduce the risk of cancer of the colon, stomach, mouth, throat, esophagus, lungs, pancreas, and bladder, as well as lessening the risk of heart disease and stroke. Necessary proteins can be supplied by beans, soy, lentils, tofu, and vegetables.

3) *Try not to eat fatty meats – especially ground beef.* Ground beef has saturated fat mixed in with the meat so there is no way it can be separated out; the percentage of fat in ground beef is much higher than in lean meat portions with the fat trimmed away. Another important issue: many animals are fed hormones to "beef them up," and they are also often on antibiotics to combat the secondary effects of the hormones. No human needs any of these contaminants in their diet.

> ❖ ❖ ❖ ❖ ❖
> My general recommendation is to eat meat as infrequently as possible

There is growing evidence suggesting that all meats, even lean red meats, can increase the risk of colon and prostatic cancer, so if you can stay away from them altogether, it's all to the good. Red meats are all high in saturated fats – those fats that cause cancer and heart disease and elevate your "bad" LDL cholesterol while lowering your "good" HDL. Poultry has almost as much cholesterol as red meat, even if you cut away its fat and skin. My general recommendation is to eat meat as infrequently as possible. If you must eat it, cut it into small pieces and disperse it among vegetables, as in Asian stir-fried preparations. This way, you can get the flavor of the meat without the overload that comes from eating a lot of it.

By the way, a wonderful substitute for a hamburger is a veggie burger or tofu burger. Another meat substitute is seitan – wheat gluten – which can be cooked to taste like beef or ham. If you're cooking spaghetti sauce, you can prepare soy sausages or soy meatballs instead of their meat equivalents. If you refrigerate the sauce, the fat will rise to the top where you can easily skim it off and end up with a meat-free, fat-free sauce that's as good as the "real thing."

4) *Soy is invaluable.* The soybean is one of the very few plants that are a complete source of protein. It is rich in amino acids and vitamins A, E, K, and some Bs, as well as being low in saturated fats. Substitute soy for meat, and your diet will be far more healthful.

5) *Make all your snacks fruits and vegetables.* If you eat at least five to nine servings of fruits and vegetables a day, you'll be taking in the micronutrition of folic acid, potassium, B vitamins, phytochemicals, and fiber that can help reduce heart disease, cancer, and stroke. Keep a bag of peeled baby carrots on your desk, or peel a grapefruit, orange, or tangerine. Try any of the many delicious varieties of apples available today. Keep a bowl of fresh fruit salad in the refrigerator. My only caveat is that you wash the fruits and vegetables carefully before you eat them, since many come from places that don't have the strict pesticide laws we do. Furthermore, it's better if you buy organic vegetables and fruits, though they're expensive. Considerable experimentation is going on now with genetically manipulated fruits and vegetables, but we don't yet know the long-term effects of eating them. This is another reason to stick with the organically grown kind – or at least "heirloom" varieties – for the time being.

6) *Avoid pizza and other processed cheese foods.* Cheese is high in saturated fats and cholesterol and very high in sodium (about 200 milligrams per large pizza slice, to say nothing of its roughly 800 calories). If you eat pizza at all, make sure it's only once a month or so – and try to eat the kind made with low-oil, low-fat cheese, which many thoughtful pizza places have on their menus these days.

7) *Use whole grains*. They are high in fiber and micronutrients that are often depleted in our highly processed foods. Oatmeal makes a great breakfast, and a high-fiber option is always beneficial. Some people, although not saddled with a gluten allergy, do have a gluten reaction that leads to foggy-headed drowsiness and may bring on a flare-up of TN. If you're sensitive to gluten, a wheat-free, gluten-free diet for two weeks may improve your over-all health and make you less susceptible to neurologic symptoms. If it does, I would then recommend staying away from grains like wheat, rye, barley and others that are rich in gluten. The same advice applies to dairy products, which can precipitate a sensitivity reaction which can trigger trigeminal neuralgia. If you feel better without milk products, there are substitutes such as rice or soy milk and soy ice creams, cheeses and other dairy substitutes.

8) *Keep alcohol to a minimum*. Always choose one or two glasses of red wine instead of hard liquor because red wine offers the benefit of the antioxidants from the red grape skins – a benefit, of course, that you can also get from red grape juice. Women increase the risk of breast cancer when they drink large amounts of alcohol, and more than three or four drinks a day can also lead to heart disease.

9) *Don't overload on sweets.* The average 12-ounce soft drink has about 160 empty calories – no fiber, minerals, vitamins, or antioxidants. Sugar also suppresses the immune system and causes inflammation which can trigger outbreaks of TN.

10) *Substitute olive oil for butter or margarine*, and spray your cooking pans with olive or canola oil. If you do use

margarine, read the label carefully before you buy, since it may contain trans-fats and polyunsaturated fats that, when heated, break down and become highly oxidized. Unsaturated oils such as corn oil should be avoided, not only because of their trans-fats but because of their tendency to oxidize in cooking.

11) *Cut down on sodium* by going easy on prepared or refined foods. More than 75 percent of the sodium we ingest comes from processed foods. As much as possible, prepare every recipe from scratch. Steam your vegetables, and skip commercial salad dressing. Instead, mix your own vinegar, garlic, and mustard with some olive oil. Use lemon juice, and replace mayonnaise with Vegenaise, which is a tofu mix that contains no dairy products and contains no cholesterol.

12) *Drink 8 to 10 glasses of water a day.* Water flushes out the system and is the body's natural lubricant.

13) *Drink tea!* Green tea contains polyphenols that enhance the immune system and fight cancer and heart disease. But black tea is also effective, and now it seems that "white" tea may be even more effective than green tea as an antioxidant. A recent study of 3,454 people in the Netherlands found that those who drank tea daily lowered the risk of severe arteriosclerosis by 46 percent. Tea's protective effect was more evident in women than in men, though no one as yet knows why.

> ❖ ❖ ❖ ❖ ❖
> Tea's protective effect was more evident in women than in men, though no one as yet knows why.

14) *Eat cold-water fish* to make a good protein meal, especially tuna, salmon, mackerel, and halibut, which are great sources of omega-3, an essential fatty acid. Try to avoid

conventional farm grown fish, as they contain no omega 3's, are filled with antibiotics and organic hydrocarbons – a threat to trigger neurologic problems. Shrimp and lobster can also be eaten occasionally because, although they are high in cholesterol, they are also rich in protein and essential fatty acids, including omega-3. Some of the cholesterol is in the form of *phytosterol,* which can actually block cholesterol absorption in the gut. But it's worth repeating here that you should avoid older and larger fish such as swordfish or shark because of the amount of heavy metals – primarily mercury – the fish have ingested over the years as a result of toxins that have washed into our oceans. However, young ocean tuna and salmon, like their freshwater brethren, are fine sources of protein and omega-3 fatty acids. If you're a vegetarian like my wife Janie, and you don't want to eat fish, consider flaxseed oil and purslane, a weed-like vegetable eaten extensively in the Middle East and eastern Mediterranean countries. This is a delicious leafy plant, high in omega-3 fatty acids, which can be used in salad and in many other ways.

A high-fat, high-protein, low-complex-carbohydrate, low-fiber diet remains the American standard today. Although there has been a recent trend to substitute polyunsaturated fats, the proteins are still mainly from animal sources, just as most of the saturated fats are. And the carbohydrates are usually simple ones, such as fructose, glucose, lactose, and sucrose. Refined starches such as potatoes, white pasta, bagels, and other products made from white flour are the carbohydrates of choice. Fruits and vegetables – the sources of most dietary fiber – are far too few, and those that are eaten are mostly not the best choices.

SAD – sad indeed.

REDUCING FATS IN THE DIET

One attempt to rectify the Standard American Diet has been to cut down on fats and substitute polyunsaturated fats and oils for saturated fats. But this has created problems of their own. Significant reduction of fat in the diet seriously limits the intake of essential fatty acids, especially the omega-3s, which are tools for battling degenerative diseases like TN. Another problem in replacing saturated with unsaturated fats is that unsaturated fats have to be hydrogenated to make them solids at room temperature. Unfortunately, these polyunsaturated fats and transfats are susceptible to oxidation when used in cooking and baking, or in packaged foodstuffs such as doughnuts, cookies and cakes. So the addition to our diets of these types of fats often does more harm than good. For instance, replacing butter with margarine is not useful – we're just trading one bad fat for another. Only reducing both butter and margarine in our diets is a beneficial choice.

Reduction of dietary fats also reduces total dietary calories, and these calories are too often replaced by the addition of sugars. Ironically, the significant increase in obesity in the United States over the last decade has come about not because we're ingesting too much fat, but because we're substituting sugar for fat.

CHAPTER 8

The Foods We Eat

When we humans first appeared on earth, we found no industry, pollution or toxins. There were few if any contaminants in the foods we hunted and gathered. Even as recently as 100 years ago, our food sources – mainly family farms – were relatively pure. We did not need to supplement our diet with micronutrients, since nature supplied them all in the foods we ate.

But more recently, the family farm has been replaced almost entirely by agro-industry mega-farms, bringing big changes in crop management from planting through harvest. Fertilizers, pesticides and other chemicals are more widely used than ever before, resulting in serious depletion of the naturally occurring micronutrients in our foods. Fruits and vegetables are picked while still green, before they can assimilate critical minerals like magnesium. Produce is picked and stored in refrigerated freight cars for long periods of time, effectively depleting them of vital micronutrients.

Similarly, farm animal producers and ranchers have dramatically changed their methods of animal management. The liberal use of antibiotics and growth hormones has given rise to antibiotic-resistant bacteria and vitamin deficiencies in these animals. The majority of antibiotics that are produced by pharmaceutical companies are *not* sold to patients or hospitals. They are sold to livestock and poultry producers. Livestock has also suffered in the attempt to make muscles plump and streaked with fat. Grazing has been eliminated and the free-range feeders that we saw in those old John Wayne movies have been replaced by corn-fed "barn potatoes." Consequently, meats have been depleted of thiamine and other B vitamins and "good fats," but have significantly increased in the saturated "bad fats."

All these changes in the way our foods are produced have severely compromised the quality of our overall food supply. Suppliers are more concerned about shelf-life, visual appeal and controlling costs than they are about the health of those of us who consume their products. The result is that it is essential that all of us – particularly older TN patients – receive supplemental micronutrients in their diets to optimize our health.

VITAMINS AND PRESCRIPTION DRUGS

We know that certain micronutrient deficiencies can exacerbate symptoms of trigeminal neuralgia. Examples of these are vitamin B12 and the essential fatty acids found in the omega 3s and omega 6s, which can be depleted through our choice of diet, exposure to environmental toxins, medication interaction and the effects of aging. However, there are two other important micronutrients that are not related to these processes. Vitamin D is one of these.

> ❖ ❖ ❖ ❖ ❖
> A vitamin is an essential enzymatic protein that greatly facilitates the biologic processes in our bodies. Vitamins cannot be manufactured in our bodies, so they must be ingested on a regular basis in order to prevent nutritional disease conditions.

A vitamin is an essential enzymatic protein that greatly facilitates the biologic processes in our bodies. Vitamins cannot be manufactured in our body, so they must be ingested on a regular basis to prevent nutritional disease conditions. These nutritional diseases are the end result of long-standing deprivation of specific vitamins. The Recommended Daily Allowance (RDA) of micronutrients, even for healthy adults, is woefully inadequate because of deficiencies caused by interactions with medications. A good example of practical differences between RDA and ODI is in the recommendations for vitamin E. The RDA says it is 10 International Units (IU), but the ODI from many sources is now routinely 400 UI – 40 times as much!

The next chart lists some common prescription drugs and the vitamins that are depleted through their use.

DRUGS & NUTRITIONAL DEFICIENCY

This Drug causes:	Deficiency in This Nutrient:
Antacids	water soluble vitamins, ca, mg, zn, k and phosphates
Antibiotics	b2, biotin, folic acid, niacin, vit D
Captopril	zn
Cimetidine	b12, folic acid, vit D, ca, zn, iron
Cholestyramine	vit D, E, A, K, b12, folic acid
Diuretics	mg, k, zn, b2
Digoxin	mg, ca
Slo-k	b12
Sulfonylurea	thiamine
Statins	coenzyme Q10
Tranquilizers	b2, coQ10
Protonix	B12, Calcium, Vit D
Metformin	B12

MY FIVE-PRONGED
MICRONUTRITIONAL RECOMMENDATIONS

These micronutrients must – *must* – be present in our bodies at all times, and in adequate amounts, if we are to have any hope of maintaining good health. Repairs to the nervous system require even higher amounts of these nutrients:

1. *Antioxidants*: The vitamins A, C, and E, which help burn up or neutralize the free-radical oxidative stress that comes with physical and mental stress and aging.

2. *Minerals*: Selenium, magnesium, calcium and zinc, which act as catalysts in the enzymatic processes that are necessary to neutralize the oxidative stress in our bodies. Zinc is especially important to nerve health. It is a catalyst for many antioxidant enzymes, necessary in nerve sheath regeneration and *prostaglandin* production.

> **Def:** *Prostaglandin*: Any member of a group of lipid compounds that are derived from essential fatty acids. They perform crucial functions in the body, including the regulation of the workings of muscle tissues.

3. *Essential fatty acids*: omega-3 and omega-6, which decrease the inflammatory response in our bodies and also allow for less inflammatory reaction in the arterial wall. In arthritic patients, coronary patients, and some cancer patients, increasing essential fatty acids will reduce the effects of these diseases.

> ❖ ❖ ❖ ❖ ❖
>
> In arthritic patients, coronary patients, and some cancer patients, increasing essential fatty acids will reduce the effects of these diseases.

4. *CoQ10*: Formally known as *ubiquinone*; coenzyme Q10 is a compound essential for life, since it is used by every cell involved in metabolism. After the age of 50, especially if patients are taking statin drugs, CoQ10 is seriously depleted and supplements are a necessity.

5. *B complex*: To aid carbohydrate, protein, and fat metabolism.

HOW TO REPAIR NERVE TISSUE

❖ *I believe that a healthy life style, including stress control, exercise and diet with supplementation, is required to repair damaged nerve tissue.* Because of the derangements of our food sources and their micronutritional deficiencies, I believe that supplementation of vitamins, minerals, fatty acids and some coenzymes provides major benefits to TN patients.

❖ *I also believe that it is necessary to have a well-balanced diet high in complex carbohydrates such as fruits and vegetables, high in essential fatty acids, and low in the simple carbohydrates and saturated fats found in sugar and meat. Only about one-third of adults eat five portions of fruits and vegetables a day, and less than one in ten adults eat the recommended seven to nine portions. And this is in a society where medication use causes a serious depletion of some of our essential micronutrients. There is a big difference between not only the supplements chosen but the frequency and dosage at which they are prescribed when looking at these two situations.*

SUPPLEMENTATION

Assuming that the foods we eat are wholesome and well-selected, it would seem redundant to add nutritional supplements to our diet. Yet there are many reasons why supplementation is necessary to health. Environmental stress such as drought can affect the ability of land to provide adequate nutrients for the crops grown on it. The soils in which foods are grown are often depleted through over-production of the very nutrients we expect to receive from those foods. Agri-corps – enormous corporate farms where single crops are raised on hundreds of acres of land – often attempt to maintain the soil's nutrients with fertilizers that fail to provide or replace appropriate nutrients.

Another reason for adding supplements is that RDAs – recommended daily allowances as published by our government – are not adequate. People who abide by RDAs have a diet that is in fact deficient in many areas.

Supplementation is a key part of nutritional therapy – a form of treatment for many conditions, including some as obvious as iron deficiency anemia and calcium deficiencies. Similarly, not all people need exactly the same amounts of all nutrients; different people assimilate nutrients with varying efficiency. Some deficiencies are medically induced, often caused by regular use of certain prescription drugs. In such cases supplementation can replace those missing nutrients.

Why – Supplementation

- ❖ Environmental stress
- ❖ Nutritional deficiencies in food supply
- ❖ Inadequacy of the RDA's
- ❖ Supplementation for therapy
- ❖ Constitutional variations
- ❖ Medically induced deficiencies

I recommend that supplements be taken regularly, and the following chart shows which supplements should be taken and in what amounts. These nutrients help to provide a base-line of nutritional health.

SUPPLEMENTS FOR GENERAL HEALTH

Vitamin A	5,000 daily
B Complex	1 cap daily
Vitamin C	1,000 mg daily
Vitamin D	2000 IU daily
Vitamin E	400 IU daily
High Potency Vitamin and Mineral	75mg daily
Niacin	640 mg, 1 cap 2 x daily
Minerals	Multi-Minerals, 2 am and 2 pm (including zinc)
Turmeric	700 – 800 mg daily
Coenzyme Q 10	100 mg daily

SUPPLEMENTS FOR TN PATIENTS

Beyond the above micronutrients recommended for general health, the Lemole Recovery Program includes an additional supplementation plan for patients suffering from TN and other facial neuralgias.

B12	1000 mg daily (not by mouth) for first week, then every 3 days, then weekly, then monthly
Alpha Lipoic Acid	100 mg, 1 cap 2 x daily
Flax Seed Oil	1 Tbsp daily
Lecithin	1200 mg daily
L-Lysine	500 mg, 2 caps, 3 x daily
NAC (n-acetyl cysteine)	600 mg 2 x daily
Omega 3 fatty acids	1000 mg, 1 cap 3 x daily
SAMe	400 mg daily
Ultra GLA	300 mg daily

SUPPLEMENTATION NOTES

❖ All supplements should be taken with meals except for amino acids such as NAC, L-Lysine and SAMe, which should be taken between meals.

❖ Although the supplements recommended for General Health in the chart above are not specific to trigeminal neuralgia, adequate levels are necessary to optimize myelin sheath repair.

❖ There is a product that may be beneficial in treating trigeminal neuralgia – Myelin Sheath Support, about which more information can be found at www. planetaryherbals.com.

❖ Since the initial event in facial neuralgias is inflammation, other antioxidants like alpha lipoic acid and turmeric have also been shown to be effective

A NOTE ABOUT GLUTATHIONE

Integrative neurologists including Dr. David Perlemutter have been using intravenous *glutathione* for neurologic conditions like epilepsy, autism and multiple sclerosis with great success. Unfortunately, oral glutathione is not well absorbed although there are new products that may be better digested. The best oral source of glutathione is NAC (n-acetyl cysteine). This amino acid is converted to glutathione when absorbed by the body. It may be beneficial to add NAC to the list of supplements for control or prevention of trigeminal neuralgia recurrence.

> **Def:** *Glutathione*: An anti-oxidant that protects cell structures from free-radicals and other products of inflammation.

Causes of Vitamin & Mineral Deficiencies

✛ Impaired absorption (drugs, allergies, leaky gut syndrome etc.)

✛ Increased Need:

◆ Dietary change (less EFA, processed food, trans fats)

◆ Drugs

◆ ⇧ Physical, mental stress

◆ ⇧ Pollution

◆ ⇧ Oxidation

FOOD PROCESSING

A century ago, 10% of our food was processed. Today, over 90% is processed. The application of milling, refining, canning, hydrogenating, and other machinations are now almost universal in our food supply. This significantly depletes most of our foods of micronutrients like vitamins, minerals, essential fatty acids, amino acids and fiber. Referring to the depletion of critical omega3 essential fatty acids, Artimis Simopoulos, M.D. (1997 chairman of the Nutrition Coordinating Committee at the National Institute of Health) said, "The admonishment to 'eat a balanced diet' makes no sense when our food has been stripped of one of its most essential nutrients." The same holds true for the 85% decrease in fiber and the loss of the other micronutrients over the past century. Processing food improves the appearance, shelf life and taste – and it does often lower the cost of the product. Unfortunately, it does nothing good for the micronutrients that were present in the food before the procedure.

Changes in the Mineral Content of Some Fruits and Vegetables, 1963-1992*

Mineral	Average % Change
Calcium	-29.82
Iron	-32.00
Magnesium	-21.08
Phosphorous	-11.09
Potassium	-6.48

*Fruits and vegetables measured: oranges, apples, bananas, carrots, potatoes, corn, tomatoes, celery, romaine lettuce, broccoli, iceberg lettuce, collard greens and chard

Processing can either be micronutrient harmful or "micronutrient neutral." For example, eating food made with flour which has been refined and stripped of its fiber of leads to the possibility of gastrointestinal disturbance, increases insulin resistance and can lead to obesity. Eating processed soups and other foods that have lost much of their potassium and magnesium –with salt substituted – can lead to hypertension and sodium overload, along with the loss of these important minerals.

The loss of micronutrients from processing food is only half the story. Added flavor enhancers such as MSG, colorings like the ever-present "red dye #2", preservatives for extended shelf life – the list of non-food substances in processed foods is practically endless, as you can tell from trying to read through the entire list of ingredients on a package label.. There have been major changes in the processing of vegetable oils, and in how wheat is processed from the hull.

Domestic Beef vs. Wild Game

Fat	+537%
EFA	-68%
Magnesium	-24%
Potassium	-19%
Copper	-61%
Manganese	-37%

There has been a huge increase in corn consumption in the United States. This shows up not so much in the processed foods sections of the grocery store, but primarily in the feeding of cattle and poultry, and in the shift to high-fructose corn syrup as the industrial food sweetener of choice, replacing ordinary sugars made from beets or sugarcane. Since corn is high in Omega 6 fatty acids, this change in our diet incorporates the Omega 6s into our cell membranes which then become stiffer, less pliable and less receptive to healthy metabolism. This also increases insulin resistance, and induces the incidence of free radicals and inflammation in our bodies. And, as you now know, it is vitally important to decrease inflammation to minimize trigeminal neuralgia symptoms.

Trans-fats – those artificial, poorly metabolized, unstable oils that are used to make cakes, breads, doughnuts and a host of other processed products – have risen to account for almost 14% of the typical American's daily diet. A century ago, they were virtually nonexistent.

It is clear that this galloping increase in processed food consumption has had a marked negative effect on our well being. It is also clear that it's up to us to "push back" against blindly accepting these food-like substances as replacements for real foods, if we are to maintain our health.

The good news is that more of us *are* making more healthful choices in our diets, replacing some meat and dairy products with additional fruits and vegetables. Organic products are much more widely available in this country than just a few years ago, with farmers' markets and mainline grocers' organic offerings increasing exponentially. This is an important development, because it is better for us to get our nutrients from natural foods rather than through supplements whenever that is possible. Researchers are finding that fruits and vegetables not only provide naturally occurring vitamins and minerals, but many other micronutrient compounds that seem to boost the effectiveness

of antioxidants. It is likely, too, that there are many more beneficial molecules in our natural food supply that will eventually be
indentified down the road – yet that makes them no less good for
our health today.

HERBS

People have been using herbs in cooking and to treat illness for thousands of years. Herbs as remedies are depicted in
Egyptian tomb paintings, and papyrus documents provide the
earliest written medical prescriptions for onions and garlic.
Adding herbs to your diet will not only improve the flavor of the
food you eat, but will add important nutrients.

Even though it was the drug industry that initially sold "natural remedies" such as quinine from the cinchona tree and digi-
talis from foxglove, you should be wary of taking herbs unless
you know the strength of the doses, since overuse can cause toxicity. Also, many of these herbs come from third-world countries
and may be contaminated with metals or sprays from the country
of origin – they're not reliably regulated when they're brought
into the U.S. Make sure you buy your natural herb supplements
from a reputable company with a good, long history of offering
high-quality products.

And now – it's time to eat!

CHAPTER 9

The Lemole Food Pyramid

A 21ST CENTURY FOOD PYRAMID

The old food pyramid is seriously out of date.

The USDA Food Pyramid[7] was designed in an attempt to illustrate what foods should be included in a healthful diet, and how much of each. Unfortunately, this pyramid has some serious shortcomings, and has been controversial since it was introduced.

It makes no distinction between whole grains and refined grains, for instance. White flour breads and bagels, white rice, white pasta, and refined and processed cereals could theoretically compose the foundation of the pyramid's recommended diet, instead of emphasizing whole grains such as whole wheat, barley, oats, brown rice, whole-wheat pasta and oatmeal, or whole-grain cold cereals. This is important because we are now certain about fiber's important protective role in helping to avoid cardiovascular and other disease. The *American Journal of Epidemiology* published a study of more than 11,000 men and women showing that women who con-

> ✧ ✧ ✧ ✧ ✧
> High-fiber foods have the added benefit of being excellent sources of antioxidants and folate.

---

[7] First introduced in the late 70s in Denmark, then adopted and modified by the U.S. Department of Agriculture in 1992 as The Improved American Food Guide Pyramid, the pyramid illustrates our government's suggested daily nutrition guidelines for each category of food. It has been updated at least three times, most recently early in 2005.

In 2011, the USDA dropped the food pyramid concept entirely, replacing it with a detailed set of "Dietary Guidelines," running to 120 pages!

sumed the highest amounts of fiber had the lowest risk of developing cardiovascular disease.

In the USDA pyramid, heath-supporting beans and legumes are grouped together with meat, poultry, cheese, and dairy – all high in cholesterol and saturated fat, not to mention the added growth hormones and antibiotics in the meats. Milk, yogurt, and cheese are not specified as full fat or skim. Fats and oils at the top of the pyramid are not broken down into "good fats" (essential fatty acids, non-damaged polyunsaturated and mono-unsaturated) or "bad fats" (butter, lard, damaged processed oils, and trans-fats). In effect, this pyramid suggests that you could eat white flour bagels with high-fat cheese, milk and yogurt, meat, chicken, and eggs regularly, along with lard, butter, and heat-treated, chemically processed vegetable oils – but used sparingly!

Dairy products deserve special attention here since they have been implicated in autoimmune diseases and multiple sclerosis, which is closely related to trigeminal neuralgia and is often confused with it. The proteins Beta casein A1 and A2 found in milk have been implicated in an autoimmune process which attacks a protein that is found in the healthy myelin sheath. It is possible that this process could be one of the causes of multiple sclerosis. If this is true, it could also be true in TN, so I think it is well worthwhile for TN patients to avoid milk, cheeses and other dairy products – and that includes non-fat dairy products, which contain just as much protein as the full-fat ones.

The USDA[8] Food Pyramid isn't a bad visual aid to illustrate how much of what foods people should eat. But it's an over-simplification that doesn't do an adequate good job of giving consumers the detailed information they need to make informed decisions about constructing and maintaining a healthful diet. And it's crystal clear to me that – for the TN patient – our government's view of what constitutes a healthful diet is dangerously off the mark.

THE LEMOLE FOOD PYRAMID

Dr. William Caselli of the Framingham Heart Study stated, "Vegetarians have the best diet. They have the lowest rates of coronary disease of any group in the county." The Lemole Food Pyramid represents a plant-based, whole-food, heath-supporting diet, incorporating the best from both the Mediterranean and Asian diets. This plan is high in fiber, nutrient-dense foods and essential fatty acids, and is low in saturated fats, cholesterol and sugar. It does not include meat, damaged oils, trans-fats, or processed "empty" foods. Fish is included, because fish and fish oils have been shown to reduce the risk of cardiovascular disease and appear beneficial in preventing heart attacks.

---

[8] Just a few weeks after the USDA released its new set of "Dietary Guidelines" in January, 2011, the non-profit Physicians Committee for Responsible Medicine filed a complaint against the USDA in federal court.

The upshot of the PCRM's filing is that the USDA is failing to balance two deeply conflicting responsibilities – to promote America's agricultural interests, and to protect Americans' health.

This conundrum, says the PCRM, has led the USDA to issue dietary guidelines which completely ignore "a preponderance of scientific and medical knowledge" that includes the fact that "there is no scientific basis" for encouraging people to include meat and dairy products in their diets, which the new USDA guidelines do, as did its earlier food pyramids.

Rather than remaining mute on the fact that nearly all saturated fats in our diets come from meat and dairy, says the PCRM, the USDA should specifically single out these sources of dangerous saturated fats as targets for meaningful reduction in any sensible modern diet.

It's probably unrealistic to think that the USDA can balance its conflicting obligations in these areas. Perhaps the agency should stop pretending that it can.

CARBOHYDRATES IN THE DIET

Confusion has developed regarding carbohydrates. The consumption of large amounts of unspecified carbohydrates was supposedly the basis of a "healthful diet," once the darling program of dieters and athletes alike. The simplistic message was "push the carbs." Unfortunately the carbs being pushed were *simple* carbohydrates – white processed flour in breads, bagels, pasta and white rice. Then "insulin resistance" and "syndrome X" became hot topics. Then "carbohydrate" became a dirty word – and the next dietary message of the moment became "push the protein," even though Americans already consume excessive amounts of protein.

Research now indicates that diets high in animal protein cause calcium to be lost in the urine. The more protein consumed, the more calcium is excreted. We also know that a high protein diet contributes to cancer and kidney disease, putting chronic overload on the body's filtering system. In a vegetarian or semi-vegetarian diet, protein is more than adequately supplied by soy, other legumes, whole grains, or fish (if included). After all, four ounces of protein daily is more than sufficient for a healthful diet.

THE BUILDING BLOCKS FOR
A NEW FOOD PYRAMID

Whole grain group: At least five servings daily. Whole grains (rice, barley, wheat, oats) and their whole-grain products (whole-grain breads, whole-grain cereals – both hot and cold – and whole-wheat pastas). Some people may be hyper-reactive to gluten-rich grains, so an elimination test diet is sometimes helpful.

Fresh Vegetable Group: At least four servings daily of fresh vegetables. Eat freely and without restriction, unless individually restricted (e.g., cruciferous vegetables and thyroid disease). Include crucifers (broccoli, cabbage), orange and yellow (sweet potatoes, squash), dark leafy greens, seaweed, onions, garlic and ginger.

Fresh Fruit Group: At least three servings daily. Eat freely and without restrictions unless individually restricted (e.g., high triglycerides and diabetes). Include citrus, apples, berries, tropical (mangoes, papayas), melons and bananas.

> **Def:** A *glycemic index* is a measure of the effects of carbohydrates on blood sugar levels. A low GI is preferable to a high one, since it slows the release of sugars in foods into the bloodstream.

Note: While vegetable and fruit juices are excellent, in general it is best to eat the whole fresh fruit or vegetable for increased fiber. This way, even if the fruit or vegetable has a high *glycemic index* (carrots and potatoes), its fiber content assures a slower release of sugar.

Legumes: At least two to three servings daily. Beans, lentils, peas, soy and soy products, edamame (steamed soy beans), tofu, tempeh (soybean cake), *miso*[9], soy hot dogs, burgers, sausage, etc.

Unprocessed Nuts and Seeds: Small amounts daily – just a handful. Nuts are rich in oils and calories, so TN patients have to be careful that they don't increase inflammation by increasing their body fat. Walnuts are especially high in omega 3 oils.

Fish: Fish and fish oils reduce the risk of cardiovascular disease. Focus on eating northern cold-water fatty fish—salmon, cod, tuna, herring, sardines, etc.

---

[9] Miso is a traditional Japanese seasoning made by fermenting rice, barley or soybeans with salt and the fungus kojikin. The resulting thick paste is used for sauces and spreads, pickling, or just mixing with vegetable stock to serve as miso soup. High in protein and rich in vitamins, miso played an important nutritional role in feudal Japan. It is still widely used today in both traditional and modern Japanese cooking, and has been increasingly adopted by vegetarian cooks around the world.

Vegetable Oils: Flaxseed and extra-virgin olive oil. Never heat flaxseed oil. Use olive oil or canola oil for baking and cooking. Use only cold-pressed oil and only in small amounts.

Eggs: Several weekly if desired, as long as your cholesterol levels are normal.

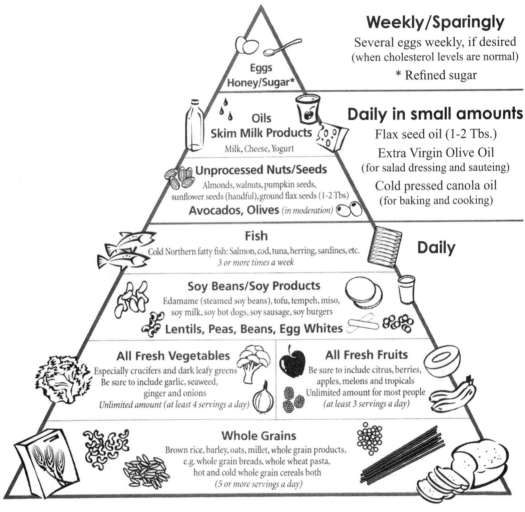

The Lemole Fish/Vegetarian Diet Pyramid

THE LEMOLE BEVERAGE PYRAMID

Liquids are a huge part of our everyday consumption, so I've added the concept of a beverage pyramid to augment the food pyramid.

Filtered or spring water is the basic liquid of a health-supporting diet. Green and white teas appear in studies to lower the risk of chronic degenerative diseases by reducing total cholesterol levels and LDL cholesterol levels, and by acting as a strong antioxidant. Green tea does contain caffeine, so if you drink 6 to 10 cups daily, decaffeinated tea is preferred.

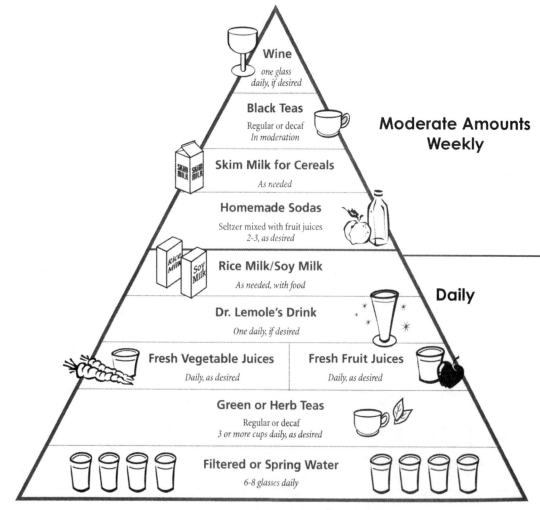

Wine
one glass daily, if desired

Black Teas
Regular or decaf
In moderation

Moderate Amounts Weekly

Skim Milk for Cereals
As needed

Homemade Sodas
Seltzer mixed with fruit juices
2-3, as desired

Rice Milk/Soy Milk
As needed, with food

Daily

Dr. Lemole's Drink
One daily, if desired

Fresh Vegetable Juices
Daily, as desired

Fresh Fruit Juices
Daily, as desired

Green or Herb Teas
Regular or decaf
3 or more cups daily, as desired

Filtered or Spring Water
6-8 glasses daily

The Lemole Beverage Pyramid

Fresh vegetable juices are excellent, as are fresh fruit juices (except for people with diabetes or high triglycerides). I also offer you Dr. Lemole's Drink, a powerhouse of nutrition, fiber and essential fatty acids in a delicious blend—a good breakfast for people in a hurry. See the recipe on the next page.

Rice and soy milk are healthful substitutes for animal milk. Homemade sodas are refreshing without the caffeine, artificial colors, phosphates, salt, and sugar or chemical sweeteners found in mass-produced soft drinks. I think TN patients should not drink very much milk – even skim, if any at all – because of the implied connection between milk proteins and myelin sheath damage. Black teas should be consumed with moderation. Wine, especially red wine, increasingly appears to offer health benefits (providing resveratrol, an antioxidant) and may be taken in moderation if desired – one glass daily.

DR. LEMOLE'S DRINK

Here's a healthy addition to anybody's nutritional regimen, but especially for those suffering with TN or related facial pain:

1 ½ cups fruit juice or coconut, rice, almond or soy milk

1 banana (or other fruits; peaches and kiwis are good)

1 Tbsp flaxseed oil

1 Tbsp powdered vitamin and mineral supplement

1 Tbsp Green Magma Plus

1 tsp lecithin granules

1 scoop whey or rice protein powder

OPTIONAL

2 tsp wheat germ

1 Tbsp nutritional yeast

Mix all ingredients and blend until smooth.

In summary, the most beneficial diet for the majority of TN patients is a high complex-carbohydrate diet, which consists of the following:

- Approximately 60 percent to 70 percent complex carbo-hydrates with little or no sugars or simple starches

- 15 to 20 percent fat, primarily unsaturated fat found in fish, flaxseed oil, monounsaturated olive oil, and canola oil

- Less than 5 percent saturated fats

- 10 to 15 percent EFAs, primarily omega-3s (and some omega-6s) derived from fish, flaxseed oil, etc.

This diet decreases levels of total cholesterol, the "bad" cholesterol LDL, the amino acid homocysteine, and body fat, while increasing EFAs. It also spares calcium and magnesium, which protect against osteoporosis, hypertension, heart arrhythmias, and other chronic degenerative diseases. A small percentage of patients who may not respond favorably to this diet will need their protein and fat increased at the expense of carbohydrates to control cholesterol, triglycerides, and sugar. I recommend getting a baseline lipid profile and blood sugar test before starting this high complex-carbohydrate diet, then stay on it for eight weeks, and finally repeat the lipid and sugar profiles. If these are still elevated, then you should consider changing to a higher-protein diet or adding supplements to lower lipid levels. Then, and only as a last resort, add cholesterol-lowering drugs.

Def: *EFA*: Abbreviation for "Essential Fatty Acids"

In the United States we've seen about a 30-percent reduction in mortality from arteriosclerosis over the last 25 years, probably due to many factors including diet, better blood pressure control, quitting smoking, increased physical activity and general health awareness, along with the advances in cardiac surgery, interventional cardiology, and medications. Often overlooked is another reason for the decrease in heart disease: more than 100 million United States residents take daily vitamin supplements, and many of our foods now contain added micronutrients – especially vitamins D and B6 and folic acid.

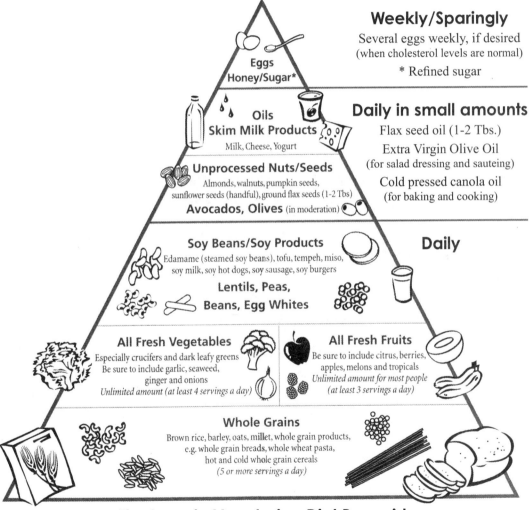

The Lemole Vegetarian Diet Pyramid

CHAPTER 10

Fourteen Day Diet

This 14-day diet is actually a plant based, good fats, high complex-carbohydrate program (with some fish, eggs and cheese) meant to jump-start my entire fitness plan.

If you're trying to lose weight, just decrease or eliminate the whole grain bread, pasta, and potato dishes.

If you want a high-protein diet, concentrate on the fish, bean and soy recipes.

The point is not to follow these suggestions slavishly, but to adapt them to your own needs.

Brand names in parentheses are simply to guide you in shopping; not all brands are available nationwide, and I am not recommending one over any other similar product.

BREAKFAST SUGGESTIONS

❖ ❖ ❖ ❖ ❖

Oliver's Oatmeal – old-fashioned oatmeal with sunflower, ground flax seeds, chopped walnuts, and cinnamon

Rice, hemp or almond milk

Honey in moderation

½ grapefruit

❖ ❖ ❖ ❖ ❖

1 boiled egg (organic DHA enhanced.)

2 slices soy Canadian bacon (Yves)

1 slice seven-grain bread, toasted if desired (with coconut oil and all-fruit spread optional)

Fresh carrot juice

❖ ❖ ❖ ❖ ❖

Flax waffles (Lifestream) with blueberries and maple syrup

Soy sausage (Gimme Lean)

Sliced papaya

❖ ❖ ❖ ❖ ❖

JAPANESE BREAKFAST

Miso soup (*pg. 94*)

Steamed brown rice

Seaweed salad

Broiled wild salmon with light soy sauce

Green tea

❖ ❖ ❖ ❖ ❖

❖ ❖ ❖ ❖ ❖

Shredded wheat – or other high fiber organic cereal

Rice, hemp or almond milk

Sliced banana

Freshly squeezed orange juice

Handful of almonds

❖ ❖ ❖ ❖ ❖

Magic Drink or Cool Green Magic Drink (*pg. 92*)

❖ ❖ ❖ ❖ ❖

Poached egg (organic DHA enhanced) on seven-grain bread

Prunes stewed in green tea and lemon slices

❖ ❖ ❖ ❖ ❖

Smoked wild salmon on whole grain bagel, toasted if desired

Low fat cream cheese, to spread lightly – 1 tablespoon

Sliced sweet onions and tomatoes, capers, and lemon

Tomato juice

❖ ❖ ❖ ❖ ❖

Tofu Scramble (*pg. 123*)

Sprouted grain toast (with coconut oil and all fruit spread, if desired)

Fresh grapefruit slices

❖ ❖ ❖ ❖ ❖

Banana nut bread muffin

Low fat organic yogurt

Sliced fresh fruit assortment

❖ ❖ ❖ ❖ ❖

Veggie Burger or non-genetically modified grain
or soy burger topped with melted cheese
(pepper jack, mozzarella, or American)

1 slice tomato

1 slice seven-grain bread, toasted if desired

❖ ❖ ❖ ❖ ❖

Flax Shake (*pg. 93*)

❖ ❖ ❖ ❖ ❖

"Less-the-Yolk" Omelet or One to Three Omelet (*pg. 83*)

Rosemary Breakfast Potatoes (*pg. 103*)

Melon slices

❖ ❖ ❖ ❖ ❖

All-Bran Buds Cereal

Rice, hemp or almond milk

Berries or banana

Freshly squeezed orange juice.

❖ ❖ ❖ ❖ ❖

LUNCH SUGGESTIONS

❖ ❖ ❖ ❖ ❖

Un-Cream of Carrot and Ginger Soup (*pg. 99*)

Daphne's Baked Tofu Sandwich (*pg. 116*)

Fruit juice soda

❖ ❖ ❖ ❖ ❖

Harry's Hummus (*pg.102*)

Pita bread for scooping

Chopped Greek Salad (*pg.107*)

Cucumber Yogurt Raita (*pg.104*)

Grapes

❖ ❖ ❖ ❖ ❖

Veggie, Soy (Boca) or grain (Garden non GMO)
burger with cheese

Toasted whole grain bread

1 Tablespoon Vegenaise, and ketchup, if desired

Lettuce, tomato, onion, pickle

French Un-Fries (*pg. 128*)

Apple

❖ ❖ ❖ ❖ ❖

Pasta and Bean Soup (*pg. 99*)

Arugula salad drizzled with extra virgin
olive oil and a squeeze of fresh lemon juice;
top with shavings of imported Parmesan cheese

Melon slices

❖ ❖ ❖ ❖ ❖

❖ ❖ ❖ ❖ ❖

Shrimp salad using Vegenaise with avocado on a bed of greens and beans with lemon vinaigrette (*pg. 111*)

Baked or fresh apple

❖ ❖ ❖ ❖ ❖

Zoe's Split Pea Soup (*pg. 100*)

Tuna salad (using Vegenaise) on romaine lettuce

Pear

❖ ❖ ❖ ❖ ❖

Blue Bell Inn Lentil Salad on baby greens (*pg. 104*)

Apple

❖ ❖ ❖ ❖ ❖

JAPANESE LUNCH

4 - 6 ounce grilled wild salmon

Edamame (*pg. 103*)

Miso soup (*pg. 94*)

Seaweed salad (Asian store)

Fresh pineapple

Green tea

❖ ❖ ❖ ❖ ❖

The Compassionate Chef's Salad (*pg. 106*)

Sliced mango with blackberries

❖ ❖ ❖ ❖ ❖

Pita Pizza—Sienna or Margarita

❖ ❖ ❖ ❖ ❖

❖ ❖ ❖ ❖ ❖

Michael's Chickpea Salad or Sandwich (*pg. 109*)

Carrot strips

Handful of raw sunflower seeds and walnuts

❖ ❖ ❖ ❖ ❖

Good Friday Soup (*pg. 98*)

White Bean and Tuna Salad on spring greens (*pg. 106*)

Clementine or orange

❖ ❖ ❖ ❖ ❖

Tofu or veggie hot dog – organic if possible

Whole grain hot dog bun (Amarillo),
chopped onions, sauerkraut, mustard,
and ketchup, as desired

French Un-Fries (*pg. 128*)

Fruit-juice popsicles

❖ ❖ ❖ ❖ ❖

Mushroom, barley and kale soup (*pg. 97*)

Sardines on seven-grain toast with
sliced fresh tomatoes

Sliced pineapple and strawberries

❖ ❖ ❖ ❖ ❖

DINNER SUGGESTIONS

❖ ❖ ❖ ❖ ❖

Festive Salmon Roll (*pg.87*)

Steamed asparagus with chopped onion
and tomato

Rosemary Breakfast Potatoes (*pg. 103*)

Sliced papaya

❖ ❖ ❖ ❖ ❖

SUMMER SUPPER

Fast pasta with fresh tomato sauce (*pg. 115*)

Garden salad with fresh herb vinaigrette

Watermelon or any fruit-juice popsicles

❖ ❖ ❖ ❖ ❖

Charlie's Tomato Sauce with "Meat Balls" (*pg. 114*)
and Spaghetti

Broccoli Baobabs (*pg. 126*)

Grapes

❖ ❖ ❖ ❖ ❖

Whole steamed or boiled artichoke with
lemon or balsamic vinaigrette

Sweet red roasted peppers with anchovies

White bean and celery salad; drizzle with a little
extra-virgin olive oil and vinegar over both

Tropical fruits, sliced

❖ ❖ ❖ ❖ ❖

❖ ❖ ❖ ❖ ❖

Stuffed Acorn Squash (*pg. 127*)

Mixed salad – greens, tomato, cucumber, onion, carrots, creamy Italian dressing

Poached pear

❖ ❖ ❖ ❖ ❖

Seared Tuna (*pg. 120*)

Christopher's Rice (*pg. 126*)

Asian Slaw (*pg. 111*)

Fresh fruit sorbet

❖ ❖ ❖ ❖ ❖

MEXICAN FEAST

Refried Bean Roll-Ups (*pg. 118*)

Spanish rice (*pg. 125*)

Salsa (*pg. 101*) and Wholly Guacamole (*pg. 102*)

Limeade – fresh lime juice with sparkling water

Melon

❖ ❖ ❖ ❖ ❖

SIMPLICITY SUPPER

Large baked white or sweet potato topped with low fat sour cream or a drizzle of olive oil or flaxseed oil (when potato skin is empty, use as a pita to wrap salad)

Spinach salad with citrus dressing and veggie bacon bits

Granny Smith or Honey Crisp apple

❖ ❖ ❖ ❖ ❖

❖ ❖ ❖ ❖ ❖

MIDSUMMER SUPPER

Baked or grilled salmon filets with
Christopher's Marinade (*pg. 115*)

Sliced peaches

Insalata Caprese (*pg. 108*)

❖ ❖ ❖ ❖ ❖

Jerry's Favorite Pasta (*pg. 113*)

Crusty rustic or peasant bread

Caesar salad (*pg. 89*)

Sliced oranges

❖ ❖ ❖ ❖ ❖

Portuguese Baked Cod with Rice (*pg. 119*)

Lima beans and corn

Green salad with olive oil, vinegar, and oregano

Sliced apples and grapes

❖ ❖ ❖ ❖ ❖

Seafood Corn Chowder (*pg. 95*)

Arugula salad

Kiwis and strawberries

❖ ❖ ❖ ❖ ❖

Don't Worry Curry (*pg. 129*)

Pan-seared tofu

Steamed brown rice with ponzu sauce (Eden)

Sautéed spinach with olive oil or garlic
and lemon

❖ ❖ ❖ ❖ ❖

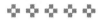

Portland Country Club's Sake-Glazed Sea Bass (*pg. 120*)

Cucumber avocado roll

Steamed white or brown rice with
sautéed shiitake mushrooms

Salad of chopped Asian greens,
Chinese cabbage, etc., with ginger dressing

Green tea

Sliced papaya with lime

Scallops, shrimp and clams over udon with
Spicy Asian Sauce (*pg. 130*)

Salad with Asian Vinaigrette

Fresh fruit sorbet

❖ ❖ ❖ ❖ ❖

RECIPES

Beverages

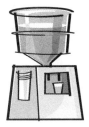

❖ ❖ ❖ ❖ ❖

STARBURST SMOOTHIE

2 cups coconut milk or coconut water or rice milk or almond milk

1 small banana or other fruit (e.g. peaches, berries, etc)

1 scoop rice protein powder

1 tablespoon ground flaxseeds

1 tablespoon lecithin granules

1/2 cup plain low-fat yogurt

Blend and enjoy. Serves 2

❖ ❖ ❖ ❖ ❖

✧ ✧ ✧ ✧ ✧

LEMOLE MAGIC DRINK

1 cup orange, grapefruit or pomegranate juice
or coconut water

1 small banana

1 cup frozen fruit
(i.e. berries, mango, papaya, etc)

1 scoop rice or hemp protein powder

1/2 tsp vitamin C crystals (Vitality C)

1 tablespoon ground flaxseeds

Blend and enjoy. Serves 1

✧ ✧ ✧ ✧ ✧

COOL GREEN MAGIC DRINK

2 cups orange, grapefruit juice or coconut water

1 kiwi

2 kale leaves

1/2 cucumber

1 handful baby spinach leaves

1/2 carrot

1/2 small lemon

1 tablespoon Green Magma Plus

Optional: 1/2 cup ice if cold drink desired.

Blend and enjoy. Serves 2

✧ ✧ ✧ ✧ ✧

❖ ❖ ❖ ❖ ❖

FRUIT JUICE SODAS

Add fruit juice – cranberry juice, lime, orange, grapefruit, etc. – to sparkling water. Garnish with a piece of fruit. Use a natural sweetener, Stevia, if more sweetness is desired.

❖ ❖ ❖ ❖ ❖

FLAX SHAKE

2 cup vanilla rice, hemp or almond milk

2 tablespoons ground flax seeds

½ banana, or any desired fruit
(pears, strawberries, kiwis, etc.)

Place all ingredients in blender and blend until smooth.
Makes 1 shake

❖ ❖ ❖ ❖ ❖

Soups

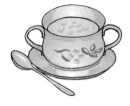

❖ ❖ ❖ ❖ ❖

MISO SOUP

> 4 cups dashi (see recipe below)
>
> ¼ cup mellow white miso
> (may use a variety of miso)
>
> ¼ pound silken tofu diced into small cubes
>
> 2 teaspoons wakame flakes
>
> 2 scallions, chopped fine

Bring dashi to boil. Remove from heat. Pour ½ cup dashi into small bowl. Add miso and mix thoroughly. Add to saucepan with tofu and wakame. Do not boil. Ladle into bowls and sprinkle with chopped scallions. Serves 4

NOTE: For vegetarian miso soup, make shiitake mushroom stock and use in place of dashi.

❖ ❖ ❖ ❖ ❖

DASHI

> 1 ounce dried konbu (seaweed)
>
> 1 cup bonito flakes
>
> 6 cups water

Place seaweed in a saucepan with 6 cups water. Bring to boil and then simmer for 5 to 10 minutes. Remove seaweed and discard. Add bonito flakes to the broth plus 1 cup cold water. Bring to a boil and then simmer for 5 minutes. Remove from heat while bonito flakes settle to the bottom. Strain stock and discard bonito flakes. Makes about 6 cups

❖ ❖ ❖ ❖ ❖

SEAFOOD CORN CHOWDER

    1 sweet onion, chopped

    1 potato, diced

    3 stalks celery, chopped

    2 tablespoons olive oil

    4 cups water

    4 tablespoons vegetarian chicken broth powder

    1 cup corn kernels

    12 littleneck clams, washed

    15 medium shrimp, cleaned

    12 sea scallops

    1/3 cup chopped fresh cilantro, plus more for garnish

    Salt and pepper to taste

Sauté onion, potato, and celery in olive oil until onion turns translucent. Add water, vegetarian chicken broth powder, and corn. Simmer for 15 minutes. Add clams, shrimp, scallops, and cilantro. Bring to boil, reduce heat and simmer until seafood is done and clams have fully opened. Add salt and pepper to taste. Sprinkle with cilantro. Serves 4

❖ ❖ ❖ ❖ ❖

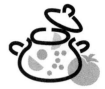

✧ ✧ ✧ ✧ ✧

CURRIED CAULIFLOWER SOUP

Used with permission from
Moosewood Restaurant, Ithaca, NY

2 tablespoons canola or other vegetable oil

1 ½ cups chopped onion

1 tablespoon minced fresh chilies,
seeds removed for a milder "hot"

1 tablespoon grated fresh ginger root

Dash of salt

1 teaspoon turmeric

1 teaspoon ground coriander

½ teaspoon ground cinnamon

2 cups cubed white or red potatoes

4 cups cauliflower florets
(about 1 medium head)

4 cups water or vegetable stock

1 teaspoon salt

¼ cup raw white basmati rice

1 tablespoon fresh lemon juice

1 teaspoon sugar

2 to 3 tablespoons chopped fresh cilantro

Salt and ground black pepper to taste

Plain nonfat yogurt (optional)

In a soup pot, heat the oil on low heat. Add the onions, chilies, and ginger and sprinkle with a dash of salt. Cover and cook, stirring occasionally, for about 10 minutes, or until the onions are translucent.

Add the turmeric, cumin, coriander, and cinnamon and cook for 1 to 2 minutes, stirring constantly to keep the spices from burning. Add the potatoes, cauliflower, water or stock, and salt, and then cover and bring to a boil. Meanwhile, rinse the rice. When the water boils, add the rice to the pot, cover, and simmer until the vegetables and rice are tender, about 15 minutes.

In a blender, purée about 2 cups of the soup and return it to the pot. Stir in the lemon juice, sugar, and cilantro. Add salt and pepper to taste.

Serve with a dollop of yogurt, if desired. Serves 4

❖ ❖ ❖ ❖ ❖

MUSHROOM, BARLEY AND KALE SOUP

> 1 medium onion, chopped
>
> 2 celery stalks, chopped
>
> 2 cloves garlic, minced
>
> 3 cups cleaned, sliced button or shiitake mushrooms
>
> 2 tablespoons extra-virgin olive oil
>
> 1 cup barley
>
> 6 cups water
>
> 4 tablespoons vegetarian chicken broth powder
>
> ½ teaspoon thyme
>
> ½ teaspoon marjoram
>
> Salt and pepper to taste
>
> 1 bunch kale, washed, stemmed, and chopped

Sauté onion, celery, garlic, and mushrooms in olive oil for 5 minutes. Add barley and sauté' 5 minutes more. Add water and seasonings. Bring to boil. Lower heat and simmer for 45 minutes. Add kale. Simmer 15 minutes longer. Serves 4

❖ ❖ ❖ ❖ ❖

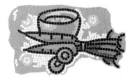

UN-CREAM OF CARROT AND GINGER SOUP

1 large onion, chopped

1 tablespoon grated fresh ginger
or finely chopped ginger root,
or to taste

1 tablespoon organic cold-pressed olive oil

3 cups organic carrots, peeled and diced

1 teaspoon mild curry powder, or to taste

1 medium potato, peeled and diced

6 cups water or vegetable stock

1 cup orange juice

Salt and pepper to taste

Chopped cilantro for garnish

Sauté onion and ginger in oil until translucent, about 5 minutes.
Add carrots and curry powder and continue to sauté for 5
minutes. Add potato and water, bring to a boil, reduce heat,
cover and simmer for about 30 minutes until carrots soften.
Then stir in juice and puree in blender until smooth. If too
thick, add more water or stock. Adjust seasoning. Garnish with
cilantro. Serves 6 to 8

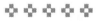

GOOD FRIDAY SOUP

2 tablespoons extra virgin olive oil

2 small zucchini, chopped

1 large potato

1 large onion, chopped

2 medium carrots, chopped

3 tablespoons chopped parsley

6 cups water or vegetable stock

2 tablespoons vegetarian chicken flavored broth
powder, if desired

Salt and pepper to taste

Place all ingredients in a soup pot and simmer for about 45
minutes until vegetables are tender. Serves 4

❖ ❖ ❖ ❖ ❖

PASTA AND BEAN SOUP

3 cloves garlic, minced or pressed

1 medium onion, chopped

3 tablespoons extra virgin olive oil

5 garlic cloves, minced or crushed

3 cups chopped fresh tomatoes or
1 (28-ounce) can whole peeled Italian tomatoes
(preferably San Marzano)

8 fresh basil leaves, chopped, plus
whole leaves for garnish

6 cups water

6 ounces pasta – broken spaghetti, elbows,
or tubetti

Red pepper flakes to taste

Salt and pepper to taste

Freshly grated Parmesan cheese

Sauté garlic and onion in olive oil. When onion is golden
and translucent, add garlic. Sauté for 1 or 2 minutes longer.
Add tomatoes and basil. Simmer on low for 10 minutes. Add
water and beans. Cook for 10 minutes. Add pasta, red pepper
flakes, salt and pepper and simmer until pasta is cooked al
dente, according to package timing. Serve in shallow bowls,
drizzle with a little extra-virgin olive oil, sprinkle with a little
Parmesan cheese, and garnish with a fresh basil leaf. Serves 4

❖ ❖ ❖ ❖ ❖

❖ ❖ ❖ ❖ ❖

ZOE'S SPLIT PEA SOUP

8 cups water

2 cups split peas, rinsed and picked over

4 slices veggie Canadian bacon, diced (Yves)

1 medium chopped onion

1 diced carrot

1 chopped potato

1 chopped celery stalk

2 chopped or pressed garlic cloves

1 tablespoon olive oil

Salt and pepper to taste

½ teaspoon marjoram

Combine all ingredients in soup pot, bring to a boil, reduce heat, and simmer gently for about 1 hour. Add more water if necessary, depending on desired thickness of soup. Serves 6

❖ ❖ ❖ ❖ ❖

Salsa, Dips and Snacks

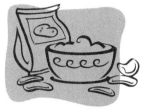

❖ ❖ ❖ ❖ ❖

SALSA

    4 large tomatoes, chopped

    1 sweet onion, chopped

    1 or 2 garlic cloves, pressed or minced

    ½ cup chopped fresh cilantro leaves

    2 tablespoons fresh lime juice

    2 fresh jalapeno peppers, sliced, or for less heat,
    use canned green chiles

    Salt and pepper to taste

If a chunky salsa is desired, chop all ingredients by hand and mix together in a bowl. If a smoother salsa is desired, put in food processor until blended. Adjust seasoning.
Makes about 2 cups

❖ ❖ ❖ ❖ ❖

✤ ✤ ✤ ✤ ✤

WHOLLY GUACAMOLE

2 ripe avocados, peeled and pitted

2 tablespoons red onion, finey diced

1 large tomato, chopped

2 tablespoons fresh cilantro, chopped fine

1 jalapeno pepper, seeded and chopped, or canned diced green chiles, or hot chile pepper sauce, all to taste

juice of 2 limes

Salt and pepper to taste

Mash avocado with a fork. Add remaining ingredients. Adjust desired hotness and seasoning. Cover lightly with plastic wrap and let flavors marry for at least an hour. Makes about 2 cups

✤ ✤ ✤ ✤ ✤

HARRY'S HUMMUS

2 cups chick peas (canned or cooked)

1 tablespoon tahini (sesame seed paste)

2 to 3 cloves of garlic, pressed or minced

1 tablespoon extra-virgin olive oil

Juice of 1 large lemon

Salt and pepper to taste

Paprika

Chopped parsley

In a mixer or blender, pure all ingredients except paprika and parsley until smooth. Put in a bowl. Sprinkle with paprika and chopped parsley. Serve at room temperature or chilled as a dip for pita bread. Makes about 2 cups

✤ ✤ ✤ ✤ ✤

✥ ✥ ✥ ✥ ✥

EDAMAME

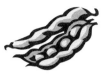

These soybeans in the pod are found
in the freezer section. Boil or steam
following package directions.

✥ ✥ ✥ ✥ ✥

STEWED PRUNES

1 green tea bag

9 prunes, pitted or not

2 lemon slices

1 cup water

¼ teaspoon sugar

Make the tea in a saucepan. Add remaining ingredients. Bring
to boil and simmer for about 30 minutes. Serves 4

✥ ✥ ✥ ✥ ✥

ROSEMARY BREAKFAST POTATOES

4 to 5 medium-size potatoes, cut into
bite-size pieces

4 tablespoons olive oil

Fresh or dried rosemary leaves, to taste

Salt and pepper to taste

Lightly oil a cookie sheet. Toss potatoes lightly in olive oil.
Sprinkle with dried or fresh rosemary, salt, and pepper. Bake at
350 degrees F for 30 minutes or until nicely browned.
Serves 2 to 4

✥ ✥ ✥ ✥ ✥

❖ ❖ ❖ ❖ ❖

CUCUMBER YOGURT RAITA

  1 cup plain or Greek yogurt

  1 cucumber, peeled, seeded and finely chopped

  2 cloves garlic, pressed

  2 tablespoons chopped fresh mint leaves

  Salt and pepper to taste

Combine all ingredients. If possible, refrigerate for several hours before serving. Serves 2

❖ ❖ ❖ ❖ ❖

Salads and Dressings

❖ ❖ ❖ ❖ ❖

BLUE BELL INN LENTIL SALAD

(Through the kindness of Chef John Lamprecht)

    2 cups French green lentils

    5 tablespoons vegetarian chicken broth powder

    5 cups water

    1 small onion, coarsely chopped

    1 stalk celery coarsely chopped

    ¼ bunch flat-leaf parsley, coarsely chopped

    ¼ cup tarragon vinegar

    1 cup light olive oil

    Salt and pepper

    Finely chopped onion, for garnish

    Hot sauce

Wash lentils and pick out any debris. Drain lentils and place in pot. Mix the broth powder and water and add to the lentils. Cover and let them soak for 1 hour. Place onion, celery, and parsley in a cheesecloth bag. Add to the lentils and stock. Bring lentils to a boil. Lower to a simmer and cook for 10 minutes or until tender. Drain lentils and let cool.

Make vinaigrette using the tarragon vinegar, olive oil, salt, and pepper. Whisk together thoroughly. Add to the lentils and toss together. Serve with finely chopped onion and hot pepper infusion or Louisiana hot sauce. Serves 4

❖ ❖ ❖ ❖ ❖

❖ ❖ ❖ ❖ ❖

THE COMPASSIONATE CHEF'S SALAD

1 head romaine lettuce

1 head leaf or Bibb lettuce

1 green or red bell pepper, cored, seeded and sliced into rings

1 tomato, sliced

1 cucumber, sliced

1 red onion, sliced

2 stalks celery, finely chopped

6 slices cheese (Mozzarella, American, or Pepper Jack) cut into strips

6 slices veggie ham, cut into strips

6 slices veggie turkey, cut into strips

OPTIONAL

2 hard-boiled eggs (sliced)

4 radishes, sliced

8 olives

Arrange artfully in a salad bowl and dress with commercial or homemade mustard vinaigrette. Serves 4

❖ ❖ ❖ ❖ ❖

WHITE BEAN AND TUNA SALAD

3 cups canned Cannellini beans, drained and rinsed

2 cans albacore tuna in spring water, well separated with fork

1 sweet onion, finely chopped

3 stalks celery, finely chopped

¼ cup extra-virgin olive oil

2 tablespoons red wine vinegar

Salt and freshly ground pepper

3 tablespoons chopped fresh parsley

1 tablespoon chopped fresh basil

Put rinsed beans in a large serving bowl. Add tuna, onion, and celery. In a small bowl, whisk oil and vinegar together and drizzle over bean and tuna mixture. Season with salt and freshly ground pepper to taste. Sprinkle with parsley and basil. Gently toss again. Serves 4 to 6

❖ ❖ ❖ ❖ ❖

CHOPPED GREEK SALAD

1 clove garlic, minced

4 tablespoons extra-virgin olive oil

1 head romaine lettuce

2 cucumbers, peeled and chopped

2 tomatoes, chopped

1 red onion, chopped

1 green bell pepper, chopped

12 kalamata olives

6 ounces feta cheese, cut into cubes

1 tablespoon fresh lemon juice

1 tablespoon red wine vinegar

Salt and pepper to taste

Press or mince garlic and add to olive oil. Chop the lettuce into bite-size pieces. Combine lettuce, cucumber, tomatoes, onions, and green pepper in a salad bowl. Add olives and cheese, dress with oil, lemon juice, and red wine vinegar. Season with salt and black pepper to taste.

❖ ❖ ❖ ❖ ❖

CAESAR SALAD

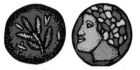

1 clove garlic

½ can anchovies

8 tablespoons olive oil

Juice of 2 lemons

Dash of Worcestershire sauce (Lea & Perrins or vegetarian)

¼ teaspoon dry mustard

1 head romaine lettuce

1 cup croutons (homemade with whole-wheat bread)

Parmesan cheese

Crush garlic and anchovies with a fork in a salad bowl. Add remaining seasonings except cheese and mix well. Add lettuce and toss well. Add croutons, and sprinkle with Parmesan cheese. Serves 4

INSALATA CAPRESE

1 head romaine lettuce

1 sliced sweet onion

1 sliced ripe tomato

6 slices fresh mozzarella cheese

6 fresh basil leaves

Salt and finely ground black pepper to taste

Extra-virgin olive oil

Arrange onion on a bed of romaine. Top with a layer of sliced tomatoes, then a slice of mozzarella. Top with a fresh basil leaf Salt and pepper to taste. Drizzle with olive oil. Serves 6

❖ ❖ ❖ ❖ ❖

CHICKPEA SALAD OR SANDWICH

  1 can chick peas (garbanzo beans)

  1 medium onion, finely chopped

  1 red bell pepper, seeded and chopped

  Juice of 1 lemon

  1 tablespoon olive oil (if desired)

  2 tablespoons Vegenaise (Follow Your Heart)

  1 teaspoon cider vinegar

  Fresh chopped parsley

  BeauMonde seasoning, to taste

  Salt and pepper to taste

Drain liquid from chick peas and rinse. In a bowl, mash beans into a paste with a fork then add remaining ingredients.

Use as sandwich filling with lettuce and tomato on seven-grain bread or whole-wheat pita or on a bed of salad greens with chopped tomato and cucumber. Makes about 3 cups or 5 sandwiches

❖ ❖ ❖ ❖ ❖

ANDEAN QUINOA & CORN SALAD

*Used with permission from
Moosewood Restaurant, Ithaca, NY*

  Grain mixture:

  1 cup raw quinoa

  1 tablespoon olive oil

  1 teaspoon paprika

  2 cups water

  1 teaspoon salt

Salad

    1 cup water

    2 cups fresh or frozen corn kernels

    2 tablespoons olive oil or other vegetable oil

    1 large onion, finely chopped (about 2 cups)

    2 garlic cloves, minced or pressed

    1 teaspoon ground coriander

    2 red and/or green bell peppers,
    seeded and diced

    1 fresh chile, stemmed, seeded and minced

    2 tablespoons minced fresh cilantro or more,
    to taste

    1 large tomato, chopped

    2 tablespoons minced fresh parsley

    ¼ cup fresh lemon juice

    Salt and ground black pepper to taste

In a sieve, rinse the quinoa under running water and set aside to drain. Heat the oil in a saucepan, add the paprika, and stir constantly for about 1 minute. Add the quinoa, water, and salt, cover, and bring to a boil. Then lower the heat and simmer for 15 to 20 minutes, or until the water is absorbed and the quinoa is tender but still chewy.

Meanwhile, bring the water to a boil in a separate pot. Add the corn and cook until tender, drain well, and set aside in the refrigerator. Heat the oil and sauté the onions, garlic, cumin and coriander until the onions are translucent, about 10 minutes. Stir in the bell peppers, chile, and cilantro, and sauté for another 3 to 5 minutes.

In a large serving bowl, combine the cooked quinoa and the sautéed vegetables and chill for 15 minutes. Stir in the corn, tomatoes, parsley, lemon juice, salt, and black pepper. Add more chopped cilantro, if desired, and serve immediately or refrigerate for later. Serves 4 to 6

❖ ❖ ❖ ❖ ❖

❖ ❖ ❖ ❖ ❖

LEMON VINAIGRETTE

1 cup olive oil

¼ cup fresh lemon juice

¼ cup white wine vinegar

1 clove garlic, pressed or minced

1 tablespoon finely chopped fresh chives

Salt and freshly ground pepper to taste

Put all ingredients in a jar. Cover and shake until emulsified. Keep in refrigerator. Makes about 1 1/2 cups

❖ ❖ ❖ ❖ ❖

ASIAN DRESSING

1 cup rice vinegar

2 tablespoons light soy sauce

1 tablespoon grated fresh ginger

1½ tablespoons sesame oil

1 tablespoon sugar

Combine all ingredients in a small bowl and whisk vigorously until well blended. Makes about 1 cup

❖ ❖ ❖ ❖ ❖

ASIAN SLAW

1 small head red cabbage, sliced or shredded

1 small head green cabbage, sliced or shredded

2 large carrots, peeled and grated

½ cup chopped scallions

¼ cup toasted sesame seeds

Dressing

> 1 cup rice vinegar
>
> ¼ teaspoon sesame oil
>
> 1 tablespoon ponzu sauce (Eden)
>
> 2 tablespoons light brown sugar

Remove and discard the cabbages' outer leaves. Shred or thinly slice and place in large bowl. Add carrots, scallions, sesame seeds, and dressing. Toss well and adjust seasonings. Allow to chill in the refrigerator.

❖ ❖ ❖ ❖ ❖

Pasta Dishes and Sauces

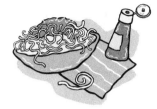

❖ ❖ ❖ ❖ ❖

JERRY'S FAVORITE PASTA

    2 tablespoons olive oil

    2 cloves garlic, pressed or minced

    8 cups fresh spinach, or 3 packages frozen

    1 pound angel hair pasta
    (whole wheat if possible)

    1 cup water

    2 tablespoons vegetarian chicken broth powder
    (optional)

    Salt and pepper to taste

Heat a pot of water for pasta. In a sauté pan, heat olive oil
and add garlic. When soft but not browned, add spinach and
continue to sauté. Put pasta in boiling water and cook following
directions on package. Add water and broth powder to spinach.
Season with salt and pepper. Simmer for 5 minutes. Serve over
pasta. Serves 4

❖ ❖ ❖ ❖ ❖

❖ ❖ ❖ ❖ ❖

MEATLESS BALLS

1 pound Gimme Lean (or substitute veggie crumbled meat)

1 medium onion, finely diced

1 clove garlic, pressed or minced

1/3 cup Italian bread crumbs

½ teaspoon dried oregano

1 egg white

Salt and pepper to taste

3 tablespoons olive oil

Put the Gimme Lean or substitute in a large bowl. Add all ingredients except the olive oil and mix together. Roll into 18 balls and brown in olive oil. Makes 18 "meat balls"

❖ ❖ ❖ ❖ ❖

CHARLIE'S TOMATO SAUCE

¼ cup extra-virgin olive oil

6 cloves garlic, finely chopped

1 medium onion, finely chopped

1 (64-ounce) can whole peeled Italian tomatoes

2 (28-ounce) cans crushed tomatoes

1 teaspoon oregano

1 teaspoon fennel powder

¼ teaspoon sugar

4 fresh basil leaves, chopped

1 teaspoon fresh chopped parsley

Red pepper flakes, if desired

Salt and pepper to taste

Parmesan cheese, if desired

Heat the olive oil in a large saucepan. Sauté garlic and onions until translucent. Add the remaining ingredients except the pasta and Parmesan.

Cook for 1 hour. Purée with hand blender. Serve over pasta and sprinkle with Parmesan cheese if desired. Makes about 15 cups

❖ ❖ ❖ ❖ ❖

FRESH TOMATO SAUCE

    4 large ripe tomatoes

    ¾ cup fresh basil leaves, shredded

    2 cloves garlic, minced

    ¼ cup extra-virgin olive oil

    Salt and freshly ground pepper to taste

Chop tomatoes. Place in a mixing bowl with basil, garlic, and oil. Salt and pepper to taste. Allow flavors to marry for 1 hour. Serve over pasta. Serves 4

❖ ❖ ❖ ❖ ❖

CHRISTOPHER'S MARINADE

    ½ cup ponzu sauce (Eden) or low-sodium
    soy sauce (Kikkoman)

    ½ cup rice vinegar

    1 tablespoon light brown sugar

    1 teaspoon dark roasted sesame oil

    1 tablespoon lemon or lime juice

    2 garlic cloves, minced or pressed

    1 tablespoon gingerroot juice
    (grated and squeezed)

Combine all ingredients. Use as a marinade. Makes about 1 cup

❖ ❖ ❖ ❖ ❖

Sandwiches, Roll-ups, Pizza and Snacks

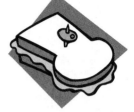

❖ ❖ ❖ ❖ ❖

OPEN-FACE BROILED FRESH TOMATO AND CHEESE SANDWICH

2 tablespoons Vegenaise

½ tablespoon chipotle salsa

2 slices seven-grain bread

4 large slices fresh tomatoes

4 slices Pepper Jack cheese

Mix Vegenaise and salsa together and spread on bread. Place 2 tomato slices on top and add the cheese. Place in broiler or toaster oven until cheese is melted. Serves 2

❖ ❖ ❖ ❖ ❖

DAPHNE'S BAKED TOFU SANDWICH

2 pounds firm tofu, rinsed and drained

2 tablespoons fresh gingerroot juice

1 tablespoon olive oil

¼ cup water

½ cup ponzu sauce

¼ cup rice vinegar

½ cup chopped scallions

2 tablespoons kudzu or cornstarch dissolved in

1/3 cup cold water

Preheat oven to 350 degrees F. Slice tofu blocks into 8 slices each. Place pieces in a lightly oiled 9 x 12-inch baking dish. Grate and squeeze ginger into a sauce pan with ponzu sauce, water, vinegar, and scallions. Bring mixture to a boil, add dissolved kudzu or cornstarch and stir until it begins to thicken. Pour mixture over tofu and bake for 35 minutes. May be served hot or cold in sandwiches.

For sandwiches, spread seven-grain bread (or your choice) with Vegenaise. Layer on large sliced tomatoes, lettuce, and baked tofu. Serves 4 to 6

VEGETARIAN CHEESE STEAK SANDWICHES

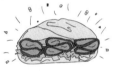

6 ounces seitan

1 medium sweet onion, chopped

1 clove garlic, minced

2 tablespoons olive oil

1 tablespoon Worcestershire sauce
(or vegetarian equiv.)

Salt and pepper to taste

3 to 4 whole wheat French rolls

4 slices provolone cheese

Sauté onion and garlic in olive oil. Add sliced seitan and Worcestershire sauce to onions. Salt and pepper to taste. Split rolls; fill with seitan mixture and top with cheese. Place under broiler until cheese is melted. Serves 3 to 4

REFRIED BEAN ROLL-UPS

1 can vegetarian refried beans

1 package all natural taco mix

1 tomato, chopped

½ cup salad olives, chopped

1 cup shredded lettuce

4 corn tortillas

½ cup shredded pepper jack

Salsa

Heat refried beans in a saucepan, add taco mix. Combine tomato, olives, and lettuce. Heat tortillas in foil or in clay tortilla pot in the oven. Lay flat and spread a layer of refried beans on top. Add vegetable mixture on half of the tortilla. Sprinkle with cheese and roll up. Serve with salsa. Serves 4

❖ ❖ ❖ ❖ ❖

MARGARITA PIZZAS

4 whole wheat pitas, split open

1 cup tomato sauce, prepared or homemade

Red pepper flakes and salt to taste

8 slices fresh mozzarella cheese

12 fresh basil leaves

Cover each pita with tomato sauce. Season with pepper and salt. Top each with 2 mozzarella slices. Broil until cheese melts. Garnish with 3 basil leaves. Serves 4

❖ ❖ ❖ ❖ ❖

Seafood Entrées

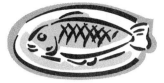

❖ ❖ ❖ ❖ ❖

PORTUGUESE BAKED COD WITH RICE

2 tablespoons olive oil

6 tomatoes, chopped

2 garlic cloves, pressed or minced

1 small onion, finely chopped

½ cup chopped black olives

2 tablespoons chopped cilantro, plus a few springs for garnish

3 pounds cod

½ cup cooked brown rice

Salt and pepper to taste

1 cup dry white wine

Preheat oven to 350 degrees F. Pour the oil into a shallow dish. Scatter half the tomatoes, garlic, onion, black olives, and cilantro in the dish. Put the fish and rice on top, season with salt and pepper and cover with the rest of the tomatoes, garlic, onion, black olives, and cilantro. Pour the wine on top. Bake for 35 to 40 minutes, basting often. Place on a warm serving plate. If necessary boil drippings to thicken and pour over fish. Garnish with cilantro sprigs. Serves 6

❖ ❖ ❖ ❖ ❖

❖ ❖ ❖ ❖ ❖

PORTLAND COUNTRY CLUB'S SAKE-GLAZED SEA BASS

8 ounces sea bass

Pickled ginger slices

1 cup sake

½ cup sugar

¼ cup juice from pickled ginger

1 tablespoon pickled ginger

Rinse and pat dry sea bass. Poke holes in the skin side with a knife.

Place a slice of ginger in each hole. Salt and pepper all sides and pan-sear in an ovenproof sauté pan.

In a sauce pan combine sake, sugar, juice from pickled ginger, and pickled ginger. Simmer and reduce by half. Let cool.

Drizzle the sake mixture over the sea bass and place in a 350 degree F oven for 10 to 15 minutes. Serves 1 or 2

❖ ❖ ❖ ❖ ❖

SEARED TUNA

2 pounds fresh tuna

1/3 cup olive oil

2 tablespoon soy sauce

¼ cup ponzu sauce (Eden)

1 teaspoon honey

½ teaspoon grated fresh ginger

2 cloves garlic

4 scallions, chopped

Cracked pepper, to taste

Cut tuna into four pieces. Combine remaining ingredients in a large bowl, and marinate tuna in the liquid for 2 hours. Heat skillet and cook tuna for 2 minutes on each side (longer if you desire). Serves 4

❖ ❖ ❖ ❖ ❖

FESTIVE SALMON ROLL

Large wild salmon fillet

2 cups cooked spinach

½ cup feta cheese

¼ cup pine nuts

Salt and freshly ground pepper

2 tablespoons extra-virgin olive oil

2 garlic cloves, minced or pressed

Remove the skin from salmon fillet. Cover the fillet with spinach, feta cheese, and pine nuts. Salt and pepper to taste. Place in baking dish that has been lightly oiled. Mix olive oil and garlic. Spoon mixture over salmon. Roll fillet from one end to the other, making a log. Tie with string in 3 or 4 places. Bake at 375 degrees F for 20 to 30 minutes, depending on desired degree of doneness. Slice from roll, removing string. Serves 4 to 6, depending on size of fillet

❖ ❖ ❖ ❖ ❖

Eggs, Tofu Scramble, and Muffins

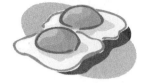

❖ ❖ ❖ ❖ ❖

"LESS-THE-YOLK" OMELET

    1 stalk celery, finely chopped

    1 red or green bell pepper, finely chopped

    1 sweet onion, finely chopped

    2 slices Pepper Jack cheese

    1 tablespoon coconut oil

    3 egg whites (organic DHA enhanced)

    Salt and freshly ground black pepper

Sauté vegetables in oil in a nonstick pan until onion is transparent. Remove from pan and set aside. Beat egg whites slightly. Heat same pan with canola oil on medium heat. Add egg whites. Cook until eggs begin to set. Add vegetables and cheese to one side and fold in half. Cover pan and cook until cheese melts. Salt and pepper to taste. Serves 1

❖ ❖ ❖ ❖ ❖

ONE TO THREE OMELET

Follow above recipe, but add 1 yoke to 3 egg whites. Serves 1

❖ ❖ ❖ ❖ ❖

❖ ❖ ❖ ❖ ❖

TOFU SCRAMBLE

1 small sweet onion, chopped

1 clove garlic, minced

½ green bell pepper, chopped

½ red bell pepper, chopped

2 tablespoons extra-virgin olive oil or coconut oil

2 pounds tofu, crumbled

1 teaspoon turmeric

2 tablespoons chopped fresh parsley or fresh cilantro

Salt and pepper to taste

Sauté onion, garlic, and green and red peppers in oil until softened.

Drain tofu. Add to vegetables and break it up with a fork to desired consistency. Add turmeric, parsley, and salt and pepper to taste. Serves 4

❖ ❖ ❖ ❖ ❖

OAT BRAN BANANA NUT MUFFINS

1/4 cup raisins

2 cups oat bran hot cereal, uncooked

1 tablespoon baking powder

¼ cup chopped walnuts

1 teaspoon ground cinnamon

¼ teaspoon ground allspice

½ cup molasses

2 ripe bananas, mashed

2 egg whites, slightly beaten

1 ¼ cups milk (rice, hemp or almond)

2 tablespoons cold-pressed organic canola oil

½ cup shredded carrot

Cover raisins with boiling water. Let stand for 5 minutes, drain, and set aside. In a large mixing bowl, stir together oat bran, baking powder, nuts, cinnamon, allspice, and molasses. In a medium bowl combine mashed bananas, egg whites, milk, and canola oil. Add all at once to the bran mixture until just moistened. The batter should be lumpy. Fold in raisins and carrot. Fill paper baking cups two-thirds full. Bake at 400 degrees F for 18 to 20 minutes or until golden. Serve warm. Makes 6 muffins

❖ ❖ ❖ ❖ ❖

Vegetable and Rice Dishes

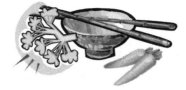

❖ ❖ ❖ ❖ ❖

SPANISH RICE

    1 onion, chopped

    1 green bell pepper, cored, seeded, and chopped

    4 tablespoons extra-virgin olive oil

    1 cup basmati rice

    1 tablespoon spicy mustard

    1 (8-ounce) can tomato sauce

    2-¾ cups water (divided)

    Salt and freshly ground pepper to taste

    ½ package taco seasoning

    3 tablespoons chopped cilantro

Cook onions and green pepper in oil. Add rice and stir. Add mustard and stir. Add tomato sauce, 2 cups water, and some salt. Bring this mixture to a boil and simmer, covered, for 30 minutes. Add more water if needed. Remove from heat when liquid is absorbed.

Sprinkle with taco seasoning and add the remaining ¾ cup water. Cook until water is absorbed. Add mixture to rice. Mix thoroughly, reheat, sprinkle with cilantro and serve. Serves 4

❖ ❖ ❖ ❖ ❖

✤ ✤ ✤ ✤ ✤

CHRISTOPHER'S RICE

  1 tablespoon cold-pressed organic canola oil

  2 tablespoons minced or pressed garlic

  1 teaspoon Asian chili paste
  (available in Asian stores)

  1 teaspoon light brown sugar

  2 tablespoons ponzu sauce (Eden)

  1 tablespoon Asian fish sauce
  (available in Asian stores)

  6 cups cooked jasmine rice

  1 cup fresh Thai basil leaves
  (available in Asian stores)

Heat oil in a wok or large saucepan. Sauté garlic until fragrant but not brown. Add chili paste, sugar, ponzu sauce, and fish sauce and stir well to combine ingredients. Add rice and basil. Stir-fry for 5 minutes until thoroughly heated. Serves 4

✤ ✤ ✤ ✤ ✤

BROCCOLI BAOBABS

  2 cloves garlic, chopped

  1/3 cup olive oil

  Red pepper flakes

  1 large head broccoli

  ½ fresh lemon

  Salt and freshly ground black pepper, to taste

Sauté garlic in olive oil until golden (not browned). Add red pepper flakes to taste (start with a pinch). Steam broccoli until light green and tender. Drizzle olive oil mixture over broccoli.

Finish with squeeze of lemon and salt and pepper to taste.
Serves 4

❖ ❖ ❖ ❖ ❖

STUFFED ACORN SQUASH

2 acorn squash, halved and seeded

1 tablespoon organic cold-pressed canola oil

1 package Gimme Lean (sausage flavor) or substitute veggie crumbled meat

1 medium onion, finely chopped

2 celery stalks, finely chopped

Salt and pepper to taste

2 tablespoons finely chopped parsley

4 tablespoons grated Parmesan cheese, or 4 slices pepper jack cheese

Place squash upside down in baking pan with a half inch of water in bottom of pan. Cover with foil. Bake in 375 degrees F oven for 30 minutes.

Meanwhile, prepare the stuffing. Heat oil in a large saucepan. Sauté the Gimme Lean until browned. Add onions and celery and sauté for 5 minutes, until softened. Season with salt and pepper and stir in parsley.

When squash are done, remove from pan. Turn squash right side up and fill with stuffing. Top each half with 1 tablespoon Parmesan cheese or 1 slice of soy cheese. Bake for 30 minutes and serve. Serves 4

❖ ❖ ❖ ❖ ❖

❖ ❖ ❖ ❖ ❖

FRENCH UN-FRIES

4 russet potatoes, scrubbed

Olive oil in a pump spray

Salt to taste

Preheat oven to 375 degrees F. Cut the scrubbed, unpeeled potatoes into French-fry size. Spray a large baking sheet with canola oil in a pump spray. Arrange potatoes without overlapping them. Spray with oil and bake for 1 hour and 20 minutes. Turn after 30 minutes and then frequently until crisp and brown. Add salt as desired. Serves 4

❖ ❖ ❖ ❖ ❖

Curry and Asian Sauce

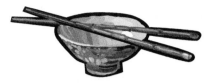

❖ ❖ ❖ ❖ ❖

DON'T WORRY CURRY

1 cup brown lentils, sorted and washed

1 cup brown rice, rinsed

4 cups water

4 tablespoons vegetarian chicken broth powder (optional)

4 thin slices fresh ginger

3 stalks celery, finely chopped

3 garlic cloves, finely chopped

1 red bell pepper, chopped

1 to 2 tablespoons curry powder, mild or hot

Salt and pepper to taste

Place all ingredients in electric rice cooker or in pot on stove. Bring to a full boil, then turn to low and simmer for 1 hour or until liquid is absorbed. Serves 4 to 6

❖ ❖ ❖ ❖ ❖

❖ ❖ ❖ ❖ ❖

SPICY ASIAN SAUCE

2 ½ cups water

2 tablespoons vegetarian broth powder

2 tablespoons ponzu sauce (Eden)

2 tablespoons black bean garlic paste

½ teaspoon freshly ground black pepper

1/3 cup cornstarch

3/4 cup water

2 teaspoons toasted sesame oil

½ cup chopped cilantro

In a saucepan combine water, vegetarian broth powder, ponzu sauce, black bean paste, and pepper. Bring to a boil, reduce heat, and simmer on low for 5 minutes.

Mix cornstarch and water in a small bowl and stir until smooth. Stir into mixture and simmer until sauce thickens. Stir occasionally. Remove from heat. Add sesame oil and cilantro. Pour over seafood with noodles. Makes about 4 cups

❖ ❖ ❖ ❖ ❖

Vegetarian Entrées

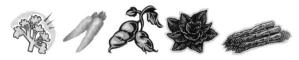

❖ ❖ ❖ ❖ ❖

HORIZONS CAFÉ – FAT-FREE SEITAN STEAK MARSALA

Through the kindness of Chef Richard Landau

½ inch dry Marsala wine, in a large skillet or wok

½ cup vegetable broth

Garlic, finely minced or pressed, to taste

Fresh herbs (rosemary, thyme, or basil)

Chopped onions or leeks

3 ounces seitan, quickly rinsed with cold water

Mushrooms

1 teaspoon arrowroot or cornstarch to thicken

Salt and pepper to taste

Preheat skillet with wine and broth to a simmer over medium heat. Add garlic, herbs, and onions. Slowly add seitan. Add mushrooms and simmer for 7 minutes or until mushrooms are tender. Season with salt and pepper.

In a separate dish, mix arrowroot or cornstarch with water until there are no lumps. Add mixture to the pan and stir. Allow to thicken, stirring occasionally, approximately 3 to 4 minutes. Serve with brown rice and steamed vegetables. Serves 1

❖ ❖ ❖ ❖ ❖

✤ ✤ ✤ ✤ ✤

HORIZONS CAFÉ – SEITAN POT ROAST

Through the kindness of Chef Richard Landau

3 ounces seitan, quickly rinsed with cold water

Baby red potatoes (small)

Baby carrots

Whole mushrooms

Sliced wild mushrooms (shiitake or Portobello)

Garlic, minced or pressed, to taste

½ cup vegetable broth

¼ cup dry white wine

Fresh thyme and rosemary

Salt and pepper to taste

Preheat oven to 450 degrees F. Place all ingredients in a large roasting pan. Cover with foil and bake for 15 minutes or until the potatoes are tender. Serves 1

✤ ✤ ✤ ✤ ✤

VEGETARIAN SAUSAGE AND ZUCCHINI SAUTÉ

1 sweet onion, chopped

2 tablespoons olive oil or canola oil

4 medium zucchinis, chopped

2 vegetarian sausages

2 tomatoes, chopped

Salt and pepper to taste

Red cayenne pepper, to taste (optional)

Sauté onion in oil until semi-soft. Add zucchini and sausage and sauté for another 5 to 7 minutes. Add tomatoes. Add salt and pepper and a dash of red pepper, to taste. Serves 4

✤ ✤ ✤ ✤ ✤

MY OWN RECIPES

_____

_____

_____

_____

_____

_____

_____

_____

_____

_____

_____

_____

_____

_____

_____

_____

_____

MY OWN RECIPES

_____

_____

_____

_____

_____

_____

_____

_____

_____

_____

_____

_____

_____

_____

_____

_____

_____

MY OWN RECIPES

_____

_____

_____

_____

_____

_____

_____

_____

_____

_____

_____

_____

_____

_____

_____

MY OWN RECIPES

_____

_____

_____

_____

_____

_____

_____

_____

_____

_____

_____

_____

_____

_____

_____

_____

_____

CHAPTER 11

Managing Stress

Not too many decades ago, the only concept most of us had of stress was in relation to bridges or buildings. Engineers use the term to describe the forces exerted on some object – say, a bridge girder. The steel from which the girder is made slowly changes in form, depending on its resistance to increasing amounts of stress. Back then, we lay people barely understood the concept of stress.

Today, stress is a part of our everyday vocabulary. "I'm so stressed out," we tell a friend. Or, "All I get at my job is stress." And it's true, because we, as well as bridges, are subjected to great forces – and it's not at all good for our health. Stress comes primarily from change. External conditions we can't control are constantly changing, and we must change accordingly. Sometimes the stresses are small – a test the next day, or shopping for tonight's meal. Sometimes they are tremendous – the death of a family member, a promotion or firing, a new relationship or rifts in an old one. As living beings we cannot avoid life, so we must recognize that the stress of change will constantly be with us.

But it's not the stress itself that affects our health; it's how we respond to it that matters. Some people actually thrive in highly stressful situations; others collapse, like a failed bridge girder, under the weight of such circumstances. And all of us differ in what kinds of situations we find stressful.

Stress can be emotional, physical, environmental or psychological. Stress can act on our bodies, our minds, our emotions and our spirits. Yet when it comes down to our physical health, stress on any aspect of our being follows the same pathway – the nervous system.

THE NERVOUS SYSTEM'S CHAIN OF COMMUNICATION

The nervous system communicates in two ways: by nerve signals passing through nerve cells and by *neuropeptides*, molecules of complex amino acids that create a response in the nervous system when secreted. These neuropeptides can stimulate emotions such as fear, pain, sadness or joy. The seat of the emotions is the mid-brain, in the area of the hippocampus, that part of the brain connected to the hypothalamus and pituitary gland. When the hippocampus is stimulated, the neurological, endocrine and immune systems are all activated; all contain receptors for the neuropeptides. These neuropeptides are like telegrams sent to coordinate individual activities and direct the body to react effectively, as a whole entity. For example, the immune cells and nerve cells "talk" to each other by means of neuropeptides.

These messages are also sent to the endocrine glands, such as the adrenal and the thyroid, which are then stimulated to secrete cortisol, epinephrine and other hormones that are vital in the "fight or flight" reaction that the body has built up over millions of years to respond to immediate physical danger. The blood-clotting system also receives these messages, since if the body is wounded it must act to stop the bleeding.

Acute stress of any kind focuses on the *medulla* – the core of the adrenal gland – which releases adrenaline. Chronic stress depletes the *cortex*, or the outer wrapping of the adrenal gland, which secretes cortisol. Adrenaline increases blood pressure and heart rate and makes the heart work faster – again, for good or ill. Cortisol suppresses the immune system and inflammation and helps regulate the utilization of glucose by the body. Chronic stress exhausts the adrenal gland and sets the body up for a depressed immune system, leading to difficulties in our handling the activities of normal life.

The whole reaction to stress is a stimulation of the sympathetic nervous system, which by nerve conduction to the adrenal glands increases the secretion of adrenaline and the release of neuropeptides. This, along with increasing adrenaline and cortisol, also speeds up the metabolism of the body, which in turn releases free radicals that cause cell damage and destruction. These free radicals then create an inflammatory condition in the body, causing the release of harmful amino acids and proteins that result in the demyelination of the trigeminal nerve, creating recurrences of trigeminal neuralgia symptoms.

The all-too-real physical dangers our cave-man ancestors faced have mostly been replaced by perceived dangers – "psychological dangers," we might call them, but they are no less real, and their effects on our bodies are just as serious.

It is well known that psychological and emotional stress can lead to high blood pressure, chest pain, heart attacks and death. It is also known that mental stress and excitation can trigger TN and other neurologic symptoms. In a study of 680 Japanese children watching a provocative television program called "Pocket Monster," their muscles and nerves became more excitable. Others who listened to a quiet program of classical music showed no such fluctuations.

> ❖ ❖ ❖ ❖ ❖
> Mental stress and excitation can trigger TN symptoms.

Among the stresses that can produce flare-ups of trigeminal neuralgia are bereavement and social isolation. People living alone without the support of family, friends or peer groups are at far greater risk of disease than those whose lives are full – no matter at what age. Job stress is a huge factor in illness, although it is more likely to be dissatisfaction with the job than job pressure that is so harmful. Dr. Susan Kobasa identified the job qualities that offer protection against morbidity and mortality in the job setting. She calls them "the three Cs":

1) Control and personal decision making

2) Challenge – a feeling of personal growth and knowledge

3) Commitment – both to the job and to life outside the job

These three attributes improve the chances of avoiding job-induced illness or death.

That the brain and the body are intrinsically linked, and not only in stress-related circumstances, is perhaps shown most vividly in the "nocebo effect" in which negative outcomes result from a harmless pill – the opposite of the well-known "placebo effect." In a British cancer group study, a cohort of patients were given placebos but were led to believe that they were actually undergoing chemotherapy. Thirty percent suffered hair loss, and fifty percent were stricken with nausea and vomiting.

Depression can be an effect of stress or a cause of stress. In either case it is a serious health problem. Hatred, resentment, bitterness, feelings of unfairness and persecution – all these are causes of stress if they are experienced over protracted periods. All cause significant chemical and hormonal changes in the body, and all may well be precursors of disease.

STRESS MANAGEMENT IN TRIGEMINAL NEURALGIA

Stress management is frequently played down or completely overlooked in therapy for TN. Usually, patients either deny their stress or say it is so common in life that it is unmanageable. Others feel that they can control the stress in their lives through their own initiative. Integrating stress management into a TN program is essential, since there is as much free-radical production resulting from mental stress as there is from physical stress. Remember oxidative stress from earlier in this book? Well, both mental and physical stress can actually cause oxidative stress and the inflammation it produces. I am among the growing number of doctors who believe that mental stress produces as much oxidative stress – and is every bit as deadly – as smoking cigarettes. Depending on the area affected, this oxidation can cause heart disease if the arteries become inflamed, cancer if the DNA becomes deranged, and neurologic disease if the nerves are attacked.

> ✧ ✧ ✧ ✧ ✧
> What happens in your life is not as important as how you respond to it.

Picture this: You have just bought a brand-new car and driven it out of the show room. While you're stopped at a red light, a car comes up from behind and slams into you. Of course, you are furious at the stupid fool behind you, but then you see in the rear view mirror a man slumped over the steering wheel. Now you are not quite as angry as you think that he might have had a heart attack. You get out of your car, walk back to check it out and – oh, no! – it's your *brother* who rear-ended you! By now, you feel no anger at all, as your concern for your brother has completely replaced it.

So it is not actually the bashing of your new car that creates the stress here. It is your negative emotional reaction to the accident that creates the pathway for stress to enter your body. The free-radical production and resulting inflammation are directly caused by your own reaction, not by the accident itself. This is the key to managing and controlling stress-induced flare-ups of trigeminal neuralgia. If you can manage your negative emotional reaction to any situation, you can minimize the physiological changes that occur from feeling negative emotions. The human brain is made up of three parts – the cortex, the mid-brain and the hind-brain. The cortex is the filter to reality. It tells me what is space and what is time, and what is happening to me in space and time. That's why I know I am standing here on the front lawn of my home on July 11th, watching my dog playing with a stick. I know this is what is happening, and that it is true – that it is actually happening, right here and right now.

The mid-brain, though, has no such idea of time or space. Any information that it receives is perceived to be real, happening here and now. The mid-brain, which contains the centers of our emotions, unfortunately perceives any negative emotions that we may feel to be real, happening here and now. This sets up the conditions for a hormonal stew, increasing glandular secretions, releasing free radicals and sending messages throughout the body to create inflammation.

Negative emotions occur in two uncontrollable places in time – the past and the future. As the old saying goes, "The past is a cancelled check; the future is a promissory note." The only "time currency" we actually have to spend is the present – the here and now. Dwelling on "If only I had…." and "What if I could…." only stirs up those free radicals all the more, and leads to increased chronic inflammation. It isn't possible to focus on the past or the future when we're concentrating on the present. That is why

> ❖ ❖ ❖ ❖ ❖
> The past is a cancelled check. The future is a promissory note.

yoga and meditation of all kinds decrease stress levels, because they keep our thoughts out of the past and the future – time zones that we can't do anything about.

There are many practices that will help you stay in the present, thinking positive thoughts and generating good feelings, and prevent your mind from straying into those useless areas of negative emotions. The important thing is to select a practice and technique that you find enjoyable. Remember, if it is not enjoyable, it will not be sustainable.

REMEDIES FOR STRESS

Overall, the Lemole Recovery Program for Trigeminal Neuralgia will help you cope with the inevitable stress life brings to all of us. There are many remedies that have proved particularly helpful in alleviating the damaging effects of stress. Many have to do with the mind, and all are meant to calm, soothe and balance the frantic pace of our lives, and to offer the peace we should try to bring into all of our days.

✤ Spirituality

I use the word *spirituality* here to mean a sense of being part of something greater than yourself, so that your existence transcends present circumstances. I do not necessarily mean a belief in God, or even just in some higher power, but rather a higher extension of obligation and opportunity above and beyond functioning only for yourself.

That spirituality is a vital component of health – an idea that continued to be "pooh-poohed" by the medical establishment as recently at ten years ago – has now been demonstrated in large-scale studies at Duke, Dartmouth, UCLA, the University of California-Berkeley, and even that bastion of traditional medicine, Johns Hopkins University. What the Eastern world has known for thousands of years, the Western world now believes.

The beneficial effects of spirituality and prayer have been shown in studies of heart disease, hypertension, stroke, cancer, inflammation of the bowel, enteritis and in many diseases of other organ systems. Even spontaneous remission has been shown to occur by altering the self-regulatory process – the positive attitude – of the individual in mind/body experiments.

We cannot, of course, make ourselves believe in something just because it will benefit our health. But in each one of us, I am convinced there is a core of spirituality that can be nurtured and made to grow. Perhaps it is enough to believe in the basic goodness and beauty of the world. It is no coincidence that so many ill people find replenishment in nature and are soothed by a forest or by the sea.

✤ Meditation

A means of relaxing the body and calming the mind, meditative practices are self-directed approaches to stilling the mind's busy-ness. They have a long history as part of the both Eastern and Western religions, but again, being religious is not essential. Meditation can be quiet contemplation of nature or of the room you sit in, or a reflection of the oneness of the universe or of the beauty of the moment.

One common meditative practice is to focus your attention and remove distracting thoughts by repeating a phrase, word or sound over and over while sitting in a comfortable position. This requires practice, but millions have achieved it and have come to rely on it for solace and support. As far back as the late 1960s, Dr. Herbert Benson, a Harvard cardiologist, studied meditation and concluded that it lowered blood cholesterol levels brought on by stress, reduced blood pressure, alleviated anxiety and chronic pain, and improved longevity and the quality of life. That's not a bad return on your investment of simply sitting quietly and meditating.

✤ Mental Imagery

Either on your own, or with the help of a prompter or guide, you can learn to affect physiological processes by imagining the outcome you desire. For instance, AIDS patients can fight their condition through imagery of "T" cells, or decrease stress through imagery of a quiet place.

Mental imagery can bring about significant biochemical and physiological changes. Through mental rehearsal – picturing a situation in your mind – you can relieve anxiety, nausea – and the pain and stress from TN.

✤ Hypnosis

A controversial means of relieving stress, hypnosis does not work with everyone, and it is a discipline full of quackery. Doctors and psychologists, not "magicians," should be selected to use it as a healing technique. Under deep trance, suggestible patients have been helped enormously, not only with stress and anxiety reduction, but in the treatment of asthma, warts, poison ivy – even the bleeding of hemophiliacs. I know first-hand of a patient who needed an operation, but could not tolerate anesthesia. He was hypnotized, the operation was performed, and the patient reported experiencing no pain. In recovery, the patient was hypnotized whenever he experienced post-operative pain – and each time, the pain disappeared. And to think that some doctors still think there is no connection between the body and the mind!

✤ Biofeedback

Techniques of biofeedback teach the voluntary control of what are essentially automatic bodily functions – blood pressure, brain-wave activity, heart rate, respiration. Yogis over the centuries have been known to slow their heart rates down to six beats per minute, and their breathing to just a few breaths per hour – not unlike a bear in hibernation.

✤ Yoga

Performed for up to an hour a day, yoga improves muscle tone, massages the internal organs, increases blood circulation, promotes deeper breathing and generally puts the mind and body at peace. When related specifically to stress reduction, it is a means of relaxation, of slowing down, and of regulating the breath – one of the key elements in my overall program. It aids chest expansion and the ability to hold your breath. It increases the vital capacity and total volume of the lungs. When we're about to go into a particularly stressful situation, we tell ourselves, "Take a deep breath…" We can do this without yoga, but the practice does help develop the capacity for breathing, which is the capacity for health.

There are many other methods of stress modification such as music therapy, relaxation response and situational reaction programs to target behavioral modification as an outcome. *Cognitive behavioral therapy* focuses on influencing behavior by changing the patient's thinking process. The beneficial effects include positive modification in relationships, smoking, medications and hostile behavior. *Laughter therapy*, popularized by Normal Cousins' best-seller *Anatomy of an Illness*, has been around for many years. Indeed, in the 17th century Sir Thomas Sydenham said, "The arrival of a good clown exercises a more beneficial influence upon the health of a town than the arrival of twenty asses laden with drugs." Laughter increases the immunity through the production of T cells and the suppression of the sympathetic nervous system. By changing the psychological environment, laughter creates an atmosphere of relaxation and calmness. Other forms of stress modification include *Ti Chi, Qigong* and other Eastern combinations of exercise and mental control, all of which help center the individual and help him stay focused in the present moment.

LOVE AND FORGIVENESS

It is becoming increasingly apparent that negative emotions are strong predictors for chronic degenerative illnesses, including trigeminal neuralgia. Positive emotions such as love, forgiveness and hope appear to help prevent these diseases and can help heal and restore health. One definition of hope is "a desire accompanied by some confident expectation of an improved outcome." In contrast, pessimism has been found to be a negative predictor of longevity and health.

The important thing is to choose a method you will enjoy and grow with it. Remember – if it's not enjoyable, it's not sustainable.

BALANCE

Balance is a theme that is particularly important in stress management. We have seen how stress, both physical and physiological, can cause disease, even though technically it's not the stress that evokes the harmful chemicals in our bodies, but our reactions to the stress. These reactions are emotional, and it is the negative emotions – fear, anger, depression and hate – that can intensify trigeminal neuralgia and a host of other chronic degenerative diseases. People who are always depressed, always angry, always afraid, always hating are at as much risk of disease as heavy drinkers or heavy smokers.

On the other hand, positive emotions like joy and love, gratitude and belonging, encourage the production of chemicals called *endorphins* that are healing in nature. We simply cannot go through life without negative emotions, and we should surely not go through life without positive ones. It is the balance between the two that we must strive to maintain, a balance based on an awareness of our position in the universe and our relationship with our own being, with each other and with all living creatures.

Today, we seem to be more impressed by human *doings* than by human *beings*. The antidote, I believe, is the realization of a wisdom outside ourselves that encourages us to be useful and kind and helpful to others. It is there where happiness lies. The keys to happiness finding us (we can never find happiness by pursuing it) are usefulness, connection (community, love) and gratitude.

Have you ever noticed that sometimes things which are not normally disturbing to you become particularly irritating, or perhaps things that usually do bother you don't seem to matter much? This is the interface between a stress and our emotional reaction to it. We can try to remove ourselves from the stress or tell ourselves that we should not be upset (even though we are), but these are generally futile efforts – and the stress just keeps building. The physical or emotional environment you are in can add to the pressure. For example, if you are overloaded and struggling with several difficult tasks and one more irritation is introduced, you might well overreact by displaying inappropriate anger, showing resentment for your "trials," or stifling anger that may be difficult to let go of later.

The emotional state that overcomes this and similar problems is called *equanimity*, commonly referred to as *balance*. Balance is the state of being centered, of realizing what is important or permanent, which gives you the ability to evaluate potentially stressful events with a clear head. It is looking at your life – and at the world – as a whole, and seeing your reaction to stress in that context. Let's say it is 2 a.m. and your 18-year-old daughter isn't home yet. You're frantic with worry until the front door slams and there she is. Now you become furious and scream at her, leaving both of you in tears. You've gone through extreme emotions – love and rage – and the stress is enormous. If only you could step back and parse the situation with a balanced outlook, you would realize you are happy and relieved that she is home, and that your anger is self-centered (she made you worry). Perhaps you'd also realize that a better reaction is possible – talking through your feelings without the rage, the tears and the stress on both of you.

This would be regaining psychological balance, but there is also physical, spiritual, and emotional balance. In the greater sense, balance pertains to centering ourselves – not only in terms of our reactions, but also in terms of our focus. Of course it is important to be focused when involved in specific act, whether at work or at home, but to tie up your life in the single-minded pursuit of a job, an avocation, a dream or a relationship can be harmful. The workaholic with a neglected family is a typical and all-too-common example.

We must balance the time we spend in work, sleep, leisure, physical activity and spiritual reflection. A well-rounded life will minimize our emotional responses to stressors. This is particularly important in negative situations, when maintaining an awareness of the world as a whole – the long view as well as the short – can restore equilibrium and perspective.

We can create a positive attitude and deal with negative emotions by:

- Seeking social support
- Laughing often
- Practicing yoga and other meditation
- Setting positive goals and making positive affirmations

- Recognizing negative self-talk and asking better questions
- Visualizing positive outcomes
- Being optimistic
- Staying balanced, or centered

Balance is vital to wellness. In any sound program for regaining and maintaining your good health as a whole, it is not enough to exercise properly, to control your diet, to manage stress effectively. All are equally important. All in combination – in delicate and beautiful balance – will ensure that the river of life keeps flowing.

CHAPTER 12

Exercise and Massage

Each of the components in my tripod of heath – diet, stress and exercise – has to be tailored considerably to meet the special physical conditions and needs of the trigeminal neuralgia patient. Significant changes in diet are required to balance the macronutrients – fat, carbohydrates and protein – as well as to supplement the micronutrients necessary to help regenerate the nerves and their sheaths. Stress is an extremely potent precipitator of TN symptoms and must be controlled. Finally, exercise – although important for total health – can sometimes trigger a recurrence of facial neuralgia symptoms.

Integrative medicine has long recognized the benefits of exercise in treating chronic degenerative disease. Regular exercise increases lean muscle mass and strength, elevates the *basal metabolic rate*, maintains weight loss, decreases resting heart rate and blood pressure, lowers low density lipoprotein and raises high density lipoprotein, increases the flow of oxygen and blood to the muscles and coronary arteries, and in general improves overall bodily functions. What a cornucopia of benefits!

Our entire society has become exercise conscious. The proliferation of health clubs, gyms, in-home workout equipment and personal trainers testifies to the fact that at least one large segment of the population is aware of the benefits of exercise. Unfortunately, another large segment is content – and often proudly and belligerently so – to remain couch potatoes.

I cannot over-emphasize how important it is to exercise regularly. Sometimes I feel like an old New England preacher when I say these things, but in my firm opinion every healthy person who does not exercise regularly is committing a sin against his or her body.

Studies in the United States and Japan show a 50% decrease in mortality and complications of coronary artery disease in patients who regularly walk compared with those who did not. Walking before eating will offset high fat meals and lower the triglycerides by 25%. However, extreme exercise increases oxidative stress and reduces the level of antioxidants – not helpful for TN patients. Unlike muscle tone and physical fitness, good cardiovascular tone requires only about 40 minutes of daily walking at a moderate 3.5 to 4 miles an hour. Choosing moderate forms of exercise is important in minimizing TN flare-ups.

Exercise is also a powerful conditioner of the lymphatic system. The role of the lymphatic system in a chronic degenerative disease such as TN is often overlooked in the typical therapeutic regimen. It is to clear from the body lipoproteins and toxic substances which contribute to chronic inflammation. Lymphatic fluid, which is larger in volume than your body's blood, is completely circulated on an average once every day. Fifty percent of the body's lipoproteins pass through the lymphatic system each day.

Exercise can increase the lymphatic flow threefold – or up to 15 times in extreme exercise – thus increasing the clearance of lipoproteins, peptides, *glycoproteins* and other messengers that may spread inflammation.

Def: *Glycoproteins* are chemical compounds made of sugar and protein that are an integral part of our tissue.

It is well known that when a physician encourages patients to exercise, compliance increases. Consider this chapter my personal encouragement to you. You can swim, walk, play tennis or participate in any number of other activities to get the exercise necessary to promote good health. The key is consistency. If you don't enjoy your exercise, you won't stick with it. Change to something else – anything that you can enjoy. The important thing is to move your body, and almost any exercise will do as long as you keep it up. Or, as they say in those commercials for a particular brand of sports clothing, "Just do it!"

EXERCISES APPROPRIATE FOR TN PATIENTS

Walking offers the advantage that no equipment is needed, other than a pair of comfortable and supportive shoes. It can be done at a steady pace, and distance can be measured accurately – either on a map or on a treadmill. Walk for 30 to 45 minutes at a pace of 3.5 to 4 miles per hour, swinging your arms freely as you go along. This will be just as beneficial as running, with the added advantage that it will put much less strain on your joints. This is especially important in trying to avoid TN flare-ups, as the bouncing movements in running can be problematic. But even patients with severe health problems can obtain an effective level of exercise just through slow and steady walking, causing minimum stress to the joints.

Swimming is another activity that is easy on the body, and is especially well-suited to people with TN. For older patients with joint problems, this is the active exercise that puts the least strain on the joints. There's no need to push yourself hard when swimming; half an hour's gentle swim is an ideal overall conditioner. Watch out for excess chlorine in public pools, as this can be a health concern.

Jumping on a trampoline or a more compact rebounder is yet another "easy-on-the-joints" exercise. I have a small trampoline in my office, and use it every day. You can start out by doing 100 jumping jacks in about five minutes, then build up the numbers to, say, 500 over a period of several weeks. This isn't for those with poor balance, of course, but even then you can get benefit from sitting on the trampoline and gently bouncing up and down. For those with active TN symptoms, this is likely a good choice.

Golf is much better exercise than most people think – especially if you walk instead of riding in a cart. Current-model push/pull carts don't require you to carry your bag, and you will walk four, five or even six miles in a typical 18-hole round. Of course, this only works well if you can avoid adding stress by being frustrated by the game – but that's just a matter of keeping yourself in balance, isn't it?

EXECISES FROM THE EAST

In addition to these traditional forms of exercise, there are other beneficial activities – most originating long ago in Asia – such as yoga, martial arts, Ti Chi and Qigong. Many of these Eastern practices have been shown to be clearly beneficial in alleviating symptoms of trigeminal neuralgia. And acupuncture, which is the ancient Chinese science of realigning the energy lines of the body, can significantly help relieve the effects of trigeminal neuralgia for some patients.

Yoga originated thousands of years ago in India as more of a spiritual practice than an exercise. The original meaning of *yoga* was "yoking together in union." Yoga was thought to enhance the link between the body and the soul, melding the two facets of the human being. There are now many and varied types of Yoga, but most focus on physical posture – taking various positions called *poses* – and on proper breathing. Yoga decreases blood pressure, heart rate, stress and anxiety, and improves muscle tone and strength, breathing, mental attitude and self-confidence.

There is plenty of evidence that yoga provides direct health benefits. In one case, after a 12-week program of practicing Yoga combined with biofeedback, one-fourth of patients were able to completely discontinue using hypertensive medications, and another 35% were able to reduce their dosage by as much as 60%. Yoga is of special value to older people because of the minimal impact yoga imposes on the skeleton.

Ti Chi is a gentle form of martial art in the Chinese tradition, most often practiced for its health benefits. It is best known to Westerners as the slow motion series of postures that groups of people practice together in parks around the world. These routines are said to help achieve harmony of the mind and body through relaxed breathing and mental focus. Psychological, respiratory and cardiovascular improvements, as well as better balance, have been documented, as have improved endurance and oxygen consumption. Ti Chi is widely practiced worldwide today, and is especially good exercise for elderly people thanks to its very low impact on the skeleton.

Qigong is an offshoot of Ti Chi, but with a greater focus on realigning the body's energy forces. It also involves a series of postures and movements reported to improve the body's energy. Qigong has been said to have a beneficial effect on the immune system, the gastrointestinal system, and chronic degenerative diseases such as arthritis, hypertension and coronary heart disease.

I hope I've made it clear that exercise is as important to your good health as any subject in this book. But there is one caveat: If you haven't been exercising and are now inspired to do so, it is wise to have a stress test prior to starting even moderate physical activity to rule out the possibility of *silent coronary disease*. Then exercise as it suits you – *just exercise*!

MASSAGE

Massage has become a common therapy – not just for athletes, entertainers and pregnant women, but for everyone. Even little babies love to be massaged – it encourages bonding, reduces crying and colic, and lulls them to sleep. Elderly adults enjoy massage as well, particularly of the back and neck muscles, and of the feet. I can think of no therapy more pleasurable, more relaxing, or more passionately anticipated.

For many years, Americans tended to overlook massage, relying instead on drugs and machines to overcome their pains and fears. But now massage has become an accepted and highly recommended medical practice. Massage would be of enormous value to anyone suffering from stress or fatigue – and that would include the vast majority of us. A recent study in the University of Miami Medical School shows workers who underwent 20-minute therapeutic massage twice weekly reported they were less tired and more clear-headed. Some employers hire free-lance massage therapists for those workers who request them, often paying much of the therapist's bills.

Massage has direct medical benefits as well. It reduces congestion and improves circulation; it increases the flow of oxygen and micronutrients to the muscles, joints and brain; it aids in the elimination of metabolic waste, it may actually cure insomnia – and it reduces pain.

Massage has been used as a therapeutic tool since ancient times. It works because the soft tissues – muscles, ligaments, tendons and *fascia*[10] – respond to touch, and most pain is felt most severely in those tissues. When applied to trigger points – those places in the muscles that evoke pain in various parts of the body – massage can reduce tightness and pain. Most headaches originate in the muscles of the neck. Abdominal and pelvic pain is usually caused by trigger points in the muscles of those regions. Lower back pain and sciatica are far more likely to come from the muscles than the vertebrae. Bad posture can misalign the muscles and bones and be a cause of constant pain. Massage – more than drugs and more than corrective surgery – can relieve pain, and I am talking about emotional as well as physical pain. In Germany, massage is routinely prescribed by doctors and paid for by insurance.

Some medical conditions – including cancer, open wounds, acute back pain, bacterial and viral disease – cannot be helped by massage. Massage in the facial area may trigger TN symptoms, so extreme caution is called for. But for everything else, including the simple rigors of daily existence, massage is a lifesaver. When massage is administered by a loving partner, it can be of enormous benefit to both parties. Mind-body therapists have proved the psychological benefits of touch. Gentle massage can communicate a profound message of love.

MASSAGE AND THE LYMPHATIC SYSTEM

Because lymphatic fluids flow, they can be affected by massage. In fact, there is a special technique – pioneered by the Danish therapists Emil and Estrid Vodder in the 1930s – that is used to stimulate circulation of the lymph called "Manual Lymphatic Drainage." MLD is a way to gently palpate and move the skin to treat the entire lymphatic system. It can be used to

---

[10] *Fascia* is a layer of fibrous tissue that surrounds muscles and bones, nerves and blood vessels and other structures in the body. It forms an uninterrupted, three-dimensional web of tissue that extends from head to toe, from front to back, from interior to exterior.

help with a variety of ailments, such as bringing down swelling and bruising, relieving sinus congestion, reducing water retention and cellulite, and easing arthritic pain. It may even strengthen the immune system.

Here are some simple massage techniques that you can perform on yourself or receive from your partner – or you might alternate roles and perform them on each other. Several of these techniques can be done at the office while taking a five-minute break or sitting on a chair at your desk.

MASSAGE TECHNIQUES

Face And Neck: Here is an exercise to make your skin firmer and help eliminate puffiness. Make sure your movements are light and soft, and begin at the neck, where many of the lymph nodes are located. Be careful as you move up above the neck, since any sensation in the facial area could precipitate a flare-up of TN symptoms.

❖ With your elbows raised at right angles to your body, place your hands as shown in the diagram. Use the middle part of your fingers to move the skin gently up and down in a circular motion, then release. Do this five times, then move your hands down an inch and perform the movement again, remembering

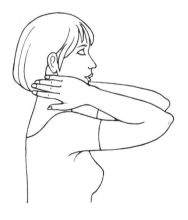

to keep your fingers straight and relaxed. Then cross your arms over your chest and work the tops of your shoulders, moving the skin forward and releasing it in a circular motion. Repeat this entire exercise a minimum of three times.

Rotary Movements (for back)

Back:

❖ Stand comfortably. With fingers pointed upward and thumbs at right angles on either side of the spine, your partner will use her palms to move the skin gently up, then toward your sides, and then release, maintaining contact so that the skin pulls the hands back. Your partner should always work up the back toward your heart. Repeat.

❖ Use the same exercise for the chest and abdomen.

Legs:

❖ Sit comfortably. Have your partner make "skin circles" around the groin area, always moving the skin toward the body. Your partner will then bend your knee, placing one hand on the front of your leg, the other behind it, as shown.

❖ Your partner will perform a "pump action" by using the front hand to softly move the skin toward the outside of your leg, then gently lift the skin upward with the palm.

✤ Then, the "scoop:" your partner will move the skin upward with a gentle scooping motion. He will alternate pumps and scoops, continuing up to the knee. Repeat a minimum of three times.

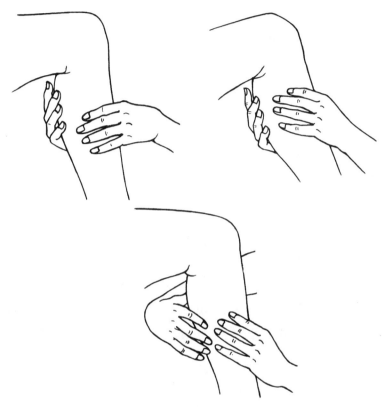

Pump and Scoop (for legs)

Note that all these exercises are used not only to benefit the skin, but also for relaxation. When your partner has finished, change places so that you become the masseuse or masseur.

SIMPLE EXERCISES TO ALLEVIATE DISCOMFORT

1. For arthritic hands, softly massage between the tendons from the knuckles to the wrist.

2. For stress, have your partner give you a back massage, with particular attention to the shoulders and

neck, which is where most tension is held. Knead as you would bread dough, then end with soft strokes for relaxation.

3. For headache, have your partner massage the back of your neck and head, then move to the forehead, the temples, and around the eyes. Make sure the massage is light and gentle. Earlier cautions for TN patients apply for all facial massage.

Calming Strokes: Stroking is the easiest of all massage techniques, and it can be as calming and beneficial as a deep massage from a professional. While there are many kinds of stroking (including "cat," "aura," "fan," "circle," "deep," and a number of Chinese techniques), all recommend an increase in pressure as you go toward the heart. The stroking needn't be heavy-handed or rough; a gentle stroking of one partner by another has been giving pleasure from the beginning of time.

We know that stroking the neck of a dog will increase its lymph flow. Overall, stroking will increase your lymph flow, and in the nicest way you can imagine.

BREATHING

Proper breathing is the most important thing you can do to maintain good health. "But I breathe all the time," you might say. "It's an unconscious process. Everybody knows that the first sign of death is when breathing stops." True enough. But if that's your reaction, you're overlooking the word "proper." There are different ways to breathe – the right way and the wrong way.

Breathing is the one essential and vital bodily function over which we have the most control. We can't direct how our kidneys or liver function, but we have the ability to master with relative ease the depth and rate of our breathing, which then affects our heart rate – and even our thinking.

"Take a deep breath," we tell ourselves before going into a stressful situation or when we want to calm down after some trauma or strenuous activity. It's an expression people have used for centuries, because we know that a deep breath will ease our mind, quell anxiety and relax our body. Quite simply – and absolutely amazingly – if you master your breath, you master your health.

If you watch young children, you'll see that they breathe from their diaphragm, that muscle that separates the upper part of our torso from the lower. As we get older, as anxiety, stress and fear creep into our lives, our breathing shifts from the abdomen to the chest, becoming more rapid and shallower. If you make the effort to shift your breathing back to your diaphragm, you will naturally begin to breathe more deeply. I urge you to make that effort.

Three easy exercises will help you breathe more deeply. Try one or two sets of all three at first, then increase the number of repetitions as you get used to doing them. If you'll do these every day – just a few minutes is all you'll need – your breathing will improve, and quite dramatically.

1. Extend your arms, touching your palms together, and take in a deep breath through your nose. As you breathe in, swing your arms out at shoulder height, ending with your body in a "T". Hold your breath for a count of four seconds, then exhale slowly, swinging your arms back in front of you, palms together again.

2. While walking, standing or just sitting, breathe in deeply to a count of four, then exhale fully to a count

of five, repeating this a few times. Do this exercise now and then, any time you happen to think of it.

3. Take a deep breath through your mouth, hold it as long as you comfortably can, then blow out as much as you can. Now, try to exhale just a little more – you can actually blow out more than you might imagine. Repeat this exercise a few times – again, just try it whenever you happen to think about it. It will slowly train you chest and diaphragm muscles to expand your lungs to a greater average volume, and help your body get used to the concept of deep breathing.

Of course, you aren't going to go through each day constantly thinking about how you breathe – you wouldn't have time for anything else. But if you will take a few minutes in the morning, in the evening and whenever else it occurs to you to do these exercises, you'll soon be taking deeper breaths as a matter of habit. It's a habit worth developing – deep breathing will absolutely, positively improve your overall health. There is no downside – unless you overdo it and hyperventilate; I don't want you fainting. Slow and steady – not quick and frantic!

TOXINS

One danger of deep breathing – of breathing at all, actually – is that we inhale the noxious chemicals that are being pumped into our atmosphere from power generation and other industrial processes nationwide. It's more difficult to find clear air anywhere in the populated parts of the world, but especially if you're a city dweller, I urge you to use an air purifier at home and at work. If you're lucky enough to live in a relatively pollution-free country environment, I encourage taking long walks. This exercise will help you clear your body of toxins and the routine metabolic waste arising from every-day life. The psychological benefits are meaningful, too – inhale clean air and your spirits will rise, clearing noxious thoughts from your mind along with such substances from your body.

YOGA

It's no accident that yoga has spread far and wide in the western world. There are now yoga studios in even the smallest towns throughout the U.S. The physical benefits of a regular yoga practice – increased flexibility, strength and stamina, along with improved posture – are balanced by the anti-stress benefits gained from the focused, mindful breathing and calm acceptance found in yoga studios of all types. Every year, more medical doctors recommend yoga to their patients, as we have recognized the wide range of benefits yoga brings to anyone who practices it regularly.

- ❖ *Breathing* – Yoga requires deep, mindful breathing, providing just the sort of overall benefits I just described in the section on breathing.

- ❖ *Flexibility* – Virtually every yoga position involves stretching muscles, ligaments and tendons, improving overall flexibility.

- ❖ *Physical control* – The physical act of getting into any of yoga's dozens of basic poses is an exercise in awareness and control of your body.

- ❖ *Relaxation* – Whatever isn't stretching in yoga is relaxing, from "relaxing into a pose" to lying flat on your back in "corpse pose." Most people have never been in a physical position that is both a stretching exercise and a relaxed condition at the same time.

❖ *Meditation* – The "still-but-focused" mind needed for meditation is a function of many yoga practices. This combination is a powerful force for wellness.

Those with facial pain conditions can easily practice yoga, although there are some poses which may not be appropriate. But those are mostly fairly advanced positions, and there are many basic poses that you can do by yourself – or in a class – that will do you nothing but good. Here are several:

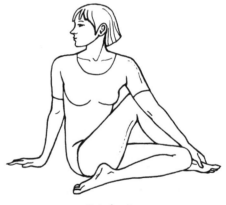

Spiral twist

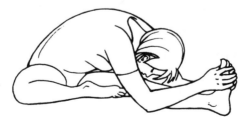

Head to knee

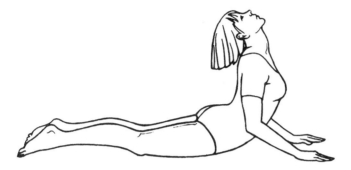

Cobra pose

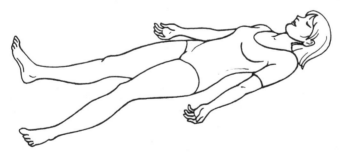

Corpse pose

Here are some "quick chair" yoga exercises you can do at work:

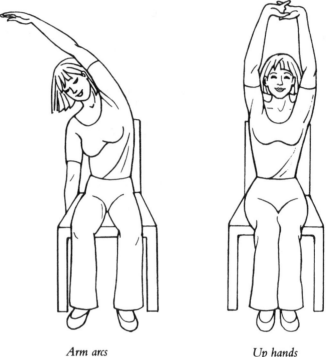

Arm arcs   *Up hands*

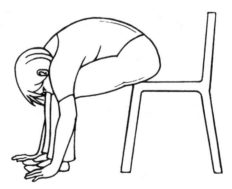

Head down

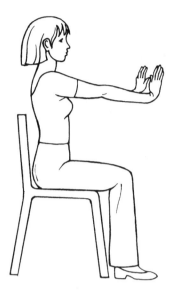

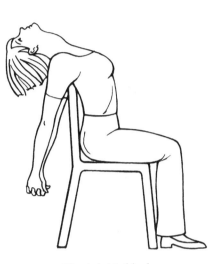

Hands in front

Hands behind back

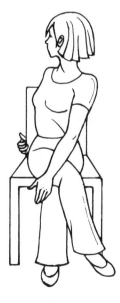

Side turns

Here are twelve basic yoga postures, or "asanas":

Sun Salutation

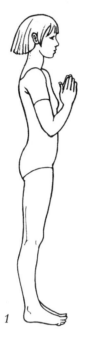

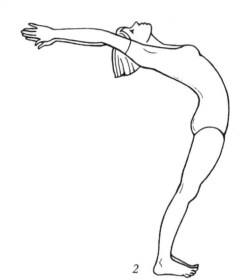

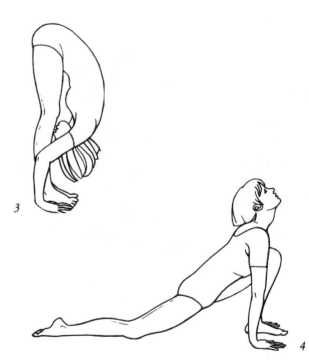

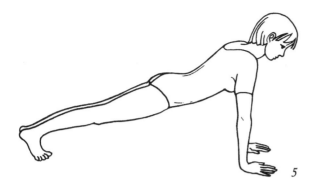

5

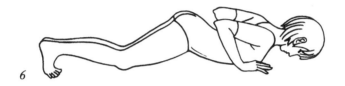

6

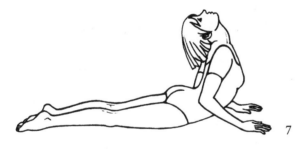

7

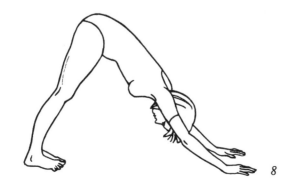

8

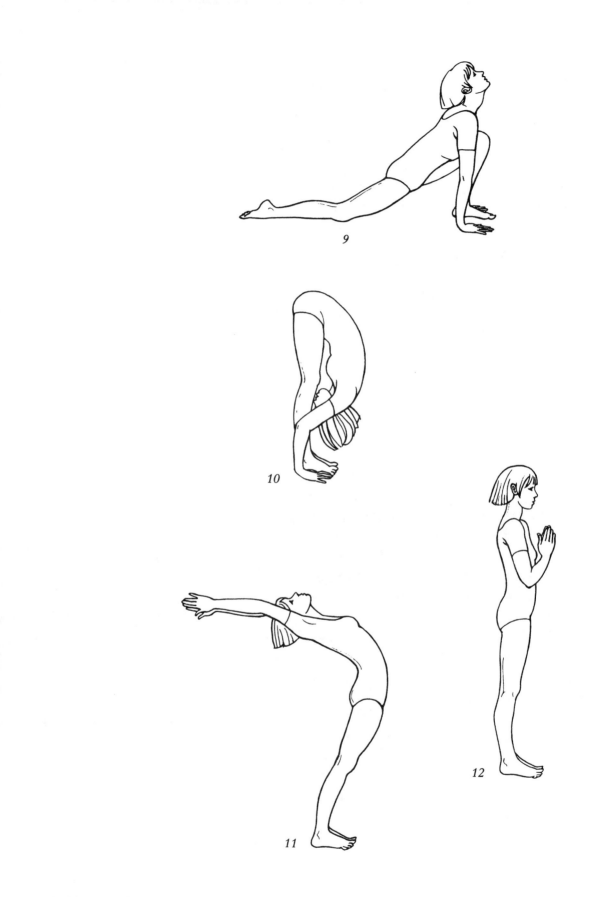

9

10

11

12

CHAPTER 13

Spirituality

"Man lives in three dimensions: the somatic, the mental, and the spiritual. The spiritual dimension cannot be ignored, for it is what makes us human."

Viktor E. Frankl, M.D.,
The Doctor & the Soul

"Stay awake and keep praying so that you won't come into a crisis. The spirit is eager but the flesh is sick."

Matthew 26:14

"This is the great error of our day in the treatment of the human body; that physicians separate the soul from the body."

Hippocrates, 377 B.C.

"Every affection of the mind that is attended with either pain or pleasure, hope or fear, is the cause of an agitation whose influence extends to the heart."

William Harvey, 1628

Integrative medicine, the kind I advocate and practice, views humankind the way Victor Frankl, the Austrian neurologist and psychiatrist, did – as spirit, mind, and body. Each of these areas has a profound effect upon the heart – my area of expertise. The terms "heartbroken" or "sick at heart" are far more than romantic metaphors; they describe a real physical condition, even though there may be no viral or bacterial cause. When the heart is at ease, it is well. When it is *dis*-eased, the spirit, mind, and body – either individually or in combination – need to be addressed.

In Western medicine the body, spirit, and mind have traditionally been segregated. Medicine's focus on the body, how its organs function and how its blood flows, ignores the physical effects of the spirit and thus creates a purely mechanistic view. To many doctors, our bodies are machines to be fixed, not people to be healed. In the seventeenth century, the French philosopher Rene Descartes concluded that there were two separate substances in the world: matter, which behaved according to physical laws, and spirit, which was dimensionless and immaterial, with an unbridgeable chasm between the two. Body and spirit; brain and mind – these were two entities that were considered to be distinct and discrete parts of human life that had to be looked at separately.

Descartes' concept dominated medical and religious thought for centuries. Western medicine does not treat the inner person, only the body; Western religion does not treat the body, only the spirit. Only now are doctors beginning to recognize the enormous role that the spirit, mind and emotions play in wellness, disease, healing – and in the maintenance of health.

While Western thought and practice remained blind to the correlation between spirit and body, societies in other parts of the world had long understood. More than 4,000 years ago in China, careful observers noticed that illness followed frustration. The Egyptians during the same period prescribed good cheer and an optimistic attitude as beneficial for health. The Greeks suggested rest and relaxation for illness, and the first-century Roman physician Galen observed that happy women had less incidence of breast cancer than those who were melancholy. In the biblical book of Proverbs, "a merry heart maketh good medicine."

William James, the pioneering nineteenth-century American psychologist and philosopher, along with Frankl in the mid-twentieth, both recognized mankind's search for a higher meaning and significance in life. "The pleasure principle might be termed the *will to pleasure*," Frankl writes. "The status drive is equivalent to the *will-to-power*. But where do we hear of that which most deeply inspires man; where is the innate desire to give as much meaning as possible to one's life, to actualize as many values as possible – what I should like to call the *will-to-meaning*?"

The "will-to-meaning," he says, is the most distinctly human phenomenon of all, since no other animal is concerned about the meaning of its existence. Yet this life force – for that is exactly what it is – is ironically overlooked by doctors whose purpose it is to maintain a patient's healthy life. Both James and Frankl understood that the body *and* the brain could be the source of sickness. They recognized a lack of spiritual fulfillment as predictive of illness; they understood the power of spirituality, the quest for life's purpose, the vital link between body and soul.

THE NEED FOR SPIRITUAL LIFE

For humankind to be centered, whole, and fulfilled, the spiritual aspect of life must play a role. Whether in the context of organized religion, in support groups without particular religious affiliation, or by following an individual path of meditation and contemplation, some form of spiritual nourishment and solace is necessary. There is empirical evidence for this statement.

Separate studies have demonstrated that prayer can facilitate healing. Others have shown that people who regularly attend church have better immune systems than those who did not. A study of patients with a religious background showed a lower diastolic blood pressure, fewer admissions to the hospital, less coronary vascular disease, and fewer complications in cardiac catheterizations than in the general population. Another study of 10,000 male civil servants in Israel showed that, independent of lifestyle considerations, religious orthodoxy alone lowered the risk of coronary heart disease.

When 230 patients over 55 years old were studied in 1995, those deriving no comfort, sustenance, or strength from religious beliefs had more than a three-fold increased mortality following open heart surgery. In 1990, another study demonstrated a significant relationship between a low incidence of cardiovascular disease and a high level of spiritual practice. In a 1991 analysis of 27 studies, 22 showed a positive relationship between health and religious commitment. Heart disease, hypertension, and overall mortality were improved by going to church.

And finally, a 1994 survey of hospitalized patients reported that 98 percent believed in God and almost as many had a conviction that spiritual and physical well-being were equally important. 75 percent prayed daily and felt their spiritual needs should be addressed by their physicians; 48 percent also wanted their physicians' prayers.

Some doctors, like my son-in-law Mehmet Oz, bring faith healers into the operating room with them; others make sure that their patients are seen by a spiritual counselor before and after major surgery. Mehmet, a Harvard-trained cardiac surgeon, started the Complementary Care Center at Columbia Presbyterian Hospital in New York, where he uses therapeutic touching, aroma therapy and hypnosis on his heart transplant and other surgical patients.

Many of the doctors at Johns Hopkins Hospital pray with their patients (including the legendary brain surgeon Benjamin Carson), and at the huge statue of Christ in its main rotunda, hundreds of religious messages are left in support of patients – not only by their families but by doctors and nurses as well.

I cite these many examples simply to show that science can be applied even to so mystical a facet of our beings as spirituality. A deep belief in some higher power or cosmological force, whether it is the God of any denomination or the simple belief in human goodness and the capacity to love, is clearly a factor in good health and rapid recovery. You must go outside yourself, see yourself in the context of the universe, be able to love, care for, and give to others. This is one important path to physical health.

SPIRITUAL HEALING

The holistic psychotherapist Daniel J. Benor defined spiritual healing as the intentional influence of one or more people on another living system without the use of any known physical means of intervention. Some individuals can, with greater difficulty, do this for themselves. Spiritual intervention, Benor says, is non-local; it is not necessarily confined to the present moment or locality. Doctors at Johns Hopkins Hospital, for instance, encourage a patient's family to set up prayer groups in their hometown while the operation is going on in Baltimore. And at Duke University, concrete evidence has been shown of the effectiveness of such distant healing.

If the patient is able to participate, so much the better. A double-blind, randomized study on the effects of prayer on coronary care patients showed that the group being prayed for required fewer diuretics and antibiotics and less ventilator assistance than the control group.

LOVE, FORGIVENESS, AND HOPE

It has long been known that negative emotions are strong predictors of heart disease and other chronic degenerative diseases. What is not so well known, but is becoming increasingly evident, is that *positive* emotions – love, forgiveness, self-esteem, optimism, hope – can help prevent disease and even restore health after an illness. In a recent study of patients who had undergone successful angioplasty, patients who scored high in positive emotions and feelings were only one-third as likely as those with low scores to have another heart attack.

You can see negative versus positive emotions at work in yourself. The next time you feel anger, hatred, or pessimism, try to become aware of your body. Your muscles will be tight, particularly in your upper back and neck; your breathing will be shallow; your stomach will churn. Quite the opposite reaction happens if you can genuinely say, "I love you," or "I forgive you," or "I have hope." Your body feels lighter, your muscles relax; your breath is deep and regular – and you're hungry!

It's more difficult to discern emotion if it has been hidden within your body, sometimes since childhood. Yet resentments fester; swallowed anger can lodge in your stomach; parental belittling when you were a child can affect your posture and self-esteem as an adult; a life scarred by unhappiness can determine the way you walk and talk and even the way you breathe. You may not be conscious of your feelings – they may be so embedded that they seem completely natural. If they're pointed out by a therapist or a friend, the response is often disbelief or denial. But the feelings are there nevertheless, and – usually with the aid of a therapist but sometimes on your own – they can be changed.

A man I know was burdened by memories of his mother – long since dead – who constantly criticized him when he was a child. He professed great love for her, said he thought of her and missed her every day, yet he walked with a stoop, his eyes were constantly downcast, he was always sick, he was unable to establish any long-term romantic relationship, and he had not lived up to his professional potential.

I advised him to see a therapist.

"Does your mother still live with you?" the therapist asked in an early session.

"Yes. She's part of me. She's in my memory, in my heart."

"Does she pay you rent?"

My friend look up, startled.

"Rent? Of course not! She's dead!"

"Well," the therapist said, "if she doesn't pay rent, you should evict her."

It was an epiphany that changed my friend's life. Evict her he did, and he finally began to live.

THERAPEUTIC TECHNIQUES

A variety of therapies designed to change emotional and spiritual outlook have become popular over the past few decades, and in each case there is ample testimony to their effectiveness.

For patients with neuropathic pain, these approaches to healing can be surprisingly helpful.

COGNITIVE BEHAVIORAL THERAPY

Cognitive behavioral therapy focuses on influencing behavior through changing the patient's thinking processes. There are beneficial effects through positive modifications in relationships, habits such as smoking, medications, diet, and hostile behavior.

MUSIC THERAPY

Clearly, there is a psychological response to music that transcends the simple pleasure of listening to it. Yet we have not been able to pinpoint exactly how music produces these complex physical and spiritual effects on the listener. It is indisputable that music calms, soothes, and inspires the spirit. For some people, it is a means of sharpening the creative urge and the imagination; for others, it encourages relaxation or stimulates meditation. Yet as Don Campbell suggests in his book *The Mozart Effect*, music can provide positive – some say amazing – health benefits as well.

"Scientists," Campbell writes, "have known that compensatory mechanisms can be triggered by loss of neurologic function. Parts of the brain that have lain dormant can 'take over,' in whole or part, the damaged function. This phenomenon may be jump-started or kicked into higher gear by music and sound, as well as by certain types of exercise and language."

Therapists at Beth Abraham, a hospital affiliated with New York's Albert Einstein College of Medicine, have shown that music is a key to gaining access to memories; that it can aid in the reversal or prevention of certain types of deafness; that it can support the recovery of neural function by promoting nerve-cell regeneration, by establishing new neural connections and pathways, and by shortening the time to recovery of neural functions.

IMAGERY THERAPY

Imagery therapy attempts to heal by evocation of the senses through the use of imagination. It's an age-old technique long used by tribal medicine men and shamans in healing rites, attempting to connect the body's movements, perceptions and emotions.

When the wife of a good friend was diagnosed with a type of brain cancer that is nearly always fatal, she went to a support group that practiced imaging – seeing mental pictures of healthy cells devouring the cancerous ones. While the imaging didn't cure her, it did provide her with enormous solace, because she felt she was actively involved alongside her doctors in battling her disease.

LAUGHTER THERAPY

In 1979, Norman Cousins wrote *Anatomy of an Illness*, which described his own miraculous cure from a life-threatening illness, primarily through laughter induced by Marx Brothers' movies. By changing the psychological environment, laughter creates an atmosphere of calmness and relaxation – far more beneficial to healing than the stress brought on by the worry and tension which usually surround illness. It delights me to think that Richard Pryor and Robin Williams may have had a greater impact on our nation's health than any number of gray-faced doctors prescribing Xansa or Percocet.

HYPNOSIS

Medical hypnosis is far different from the hypnosis practiced by magicians for entertainment. Doctors and psychologists have used it therapeutically as anesthesia and to unlock emotional inhibitions that damage the body as well as the mind. The results can be extraordinary.

TIME-SHIFTING

Time itself is often overlooked as a powerful force in healing and spirituality. Yet time has many speeds, and your relation to it must be varied based on your circumstances. To you, nine seconds may not seem long enough to accomplish anything significant. But to LeBron James, it is ample time to bring the basketball up the court, assess the defense, and then calmly make the game-winning shot. We all complain now and then about "not having enough hours in the day." But there are enough hours – and 24 is all we're ever going to get in any case – so it's actually just a matter of using them well, or misusing them. We must take and keep control of time, not let it control us. We must bend it to the needs of our psyche, not only to our material well-being.

If we can begin to dial back the pace of our ever-faster lives – jam-packed as they are with cell-calls, e-mail and the Internet – and take a little time for meditation (even just 10 minutes in the car after the commute home), for a quiet walk, for an unplanned weekend escape, our spiritual life can begin to flourish.

MEDICINE OF THE MIND

All these therapies and others have to do specifically with challenging and developing the *mind* – that part of you which can reach the realm of spiritual investigation and fulfillment – not the *brain*, which is concerned with rational thought. If your mind is calm, your body will be calm. When your body is at ease, your blood pressure, heart rate and breathing rate all decrease. And as we've explored earlier, the meditative mind cannot be in distress.

Gaining spirituality often requires a total change in mind-set. If you're frantic and rushed, burdened with work, filled with concern about your family or money or a relationship, you will have little chance to create peace of mind. Similarly, if you're angry, depressed, worried, scattered or anxious, there's no opportunity to ease the spirit. I recognize that it's a lot simpler to tell yourself to "calm down" than it is to *be* calm, but even without the aid of a therapist, there are a few ways to promote the needed change in your mind-set.

- ❖ Create a special place – a "sacred space" – in which to meditate or practice any of the other mind-altering techniques. It can be a chapel, a spacious closet, or even one corner of a room that you have mentally marked off as a quiet, safe place to center yourself and contemplate life's more profound matters.

- ❖ Think optimistically rather than pessimistically. The deal *will* go through. The relationship *will* endure. Your children *will* get over it (whatever "it" is). If you make optimism your mantra, it will in time become second nature – part of your psychic makeup.

- ❖ Be positive. This is the key to optimism, of course, a way of looking at a task or event in the best possible light. The simple attitude "I can *do* it!" is at least as important to success (and I don't mean only material success) as careful planning.

- Set positive goals – again, not only in the realm of material goods. Many people lead their lives and arrange their thoughts simply to avoid failure – the negative approach. They may well not fail – but this attitude is surely no path to achieving success.

- Practice positive visualization. I've talked already about visualization as a factor in healing. But it can also be used by the healthy to further the achievement of goals and as an aid to optimism. If you set a definite positive goal for the future (a new house in five years; a better balance in family life; a solid relationship with God), it will come to pass if you can almost actually see it already (the house with rooms and furniture, the family sits together at dinner, your God comes to you in church). The more specific these visualizing details, the better.

- Become aware of "self-talk." Perpetual use of the *"I"* word can lead to a self-involvement that excludes others from your thoughts. Narcissism virtually guarantees small-mindedness, for it limits the world to yourself and makes it impossible to think of others. The self-involved are rarely engaged in higher concepts and ideals, and certainly not with spirituality, which presupposes a force far greater than self.

- Ask meaningful questions – ones that challenge your assumptions, respect opposing viewpoints and help to broaden your knowledge. Ask questions about the "why?" of things, your relationship to the Grand Design – metaphysical questions that mankind has been struggling with since the dawn of thought. These questions are the paving stones on the spiritual road. They lead, in the Buddhist sense, to Enlightenment.

❖ Laugh. As Norman Cousins did, you can watch funny movies, listen to comedy routines, tell and enjoy jokes. But mishaps can also be funny. The ability to laugh at yourself is a rare and valuable asset. Life is at once sublime and ridiculous, and an ironic attitude is often more healing than a sentimental one. God gave us laughter, and we should use it to the fullest.

THE "NEW AGE" DOCTOR

I am one of the many physicians who now believes in both orthodox medicine – indeed, we are now at the point where much of it has become an exact science – and in integrative medicine. As I read over this chapter, I'm struck by what the medical establishment might have thought of this approach as recently as five years ago. But "New Age" medical thinking – a misnomer if there ever was one, since these ideas were propounded in Asia even before Egyptian civilization was born – has joined with scientific thinking, and spirituality has become linked with up-to-date medical technology.

Remember that the ideal healing concept incorporates the wisdom of the ancient East into the know-how of modern Western science. This is as it should be, and it arrives none too soon.

PART THREE:

The Nutrition and Science
of Facial Pain

CHAPTER 14

ORTHOMOLECULAR SCIENCE

The term *orthomolecular* was first used in 1968 by Nobel Prize Laureate chemist Linus Pauling to describe the practice of preventing and treating disease by providing the body with optimal amounts of substances which are natural to the body. Orthomolecular science aims at restoring the optimum ecological environment for the body's cells by correcting imbalances

> **Def:** *Orthomolecular science* attempts to restore the optimum ecological environment for the body's cells by correcting imbalances or deficiencies on the molecular level.

or deficiencies on the molecular level. It makes use of such substances as vitamins and minerals, fatty acids, amino acids, hormones and enzymes. It is a principle precept of orthomolecular science that genetic factors are central contributors to the biochemical environment, and that by providing the necessary building blocks such as enzymes and minerals, one can boost the reparative process – or at least prevent excessive nerve demyelination.

THE IMPORTANCE OF VITAMIN B12

Building upon the work done by Dr. Pauling, Abram Hoffer, M.D., PhD, developed treatments based on high doses of certain B vitamins and published his findings together with Morton Walker, D.P.M., in 1978 and updated them in 1996. Dr. Hoffer showed that vitamin B12 is crucial for reparative and metabolic functions of all cells, especially those with rapid metabolism like the brain and the red blood cells. That is why a deficiency of B12 becomes apparent first in the neurologic system and then later, as *macrocytic anemia*.[10] It has also been shown that because

of the high fat content and the rapid metabolism, higher doses of B12 are needed to repair the nervous system than are necessary for maintenance or repair of other organs.

Neurological symptoms of B12 deficiency can occur long before macrocytic anemia. The official level of a B12 deficiency state is about 200 picograms per milliliter of blood. However, neurologic symptoms have been seen at higher levels – below about 500 picograms per milliliter. Indeed, a study from Tufts University's Jean Mayer USDA Human Nutrition Research Center on Aging suggested that up to 42% of Americans may be deficient in Vitamin B12. The reason for this confusion is that neurologic symptoms – such as numbness, pain, forgetfulness and insomnia – are so variable that it is sometimes difficult to firmly associate them with B12 deficiency, while macrocytic anemia is readily quantifiable.[11]

Higher levels of B12 may be required due to several other causes of B12 deficiency.

The first cause of deficiency has to do with the availability of vitamin B12 in our diet. Since all of this vitamin comes from ruminants (cattle, sheep, deer, goats) and their products (milk, cheese), it may well be that the changes in how we raise these food animals (such as feeding cattle a diet of corn and treating them with large amounts of antibiotics) may deplete the B12 that is produced in their gastrointestinal tract. Ruminating animals

---

[10] This is in contradistinction to microcytic anemia, which is a state of iron deficiency.

[11] A more accurate test is measuring the level of methyl malonic acid, which is an intermediate product that can accumulate if the B12 level is low. Elevated homocysteine levels are also found in patients deficient in B12.

do not manufacture B12 themselves. It is made by the bacteria in their gastrointestinal system, and is then absorbed from the intestine by the animal. If the bacterial flora is changed by altering the diet and adding antibiotics, this may well depress the animal's levels of B12.

The use of prophylactic antibiotics in our meat supply may have consequences other than vitamin deficiencies. A study of more than 200 swine by the University of Iowa showed that 70% of them were infected with *MRSA*. After examining 20 farmers that worked with these pigs, researchers found that half of the *humans* were also culture-positive for MRSA. The majority of the antibiotics that are sold in the United

> **Def:** *Methicillin-resistant Staphylococcus aureus* is any strain of Staph bacteria that has developed resistance to antibiotics. Responsible for several difficult-to-treat infections in humans, MRSA is increasingly troublesome in farm animals as well.

States are used on cattle, poultry and domestic animals, not on humans. I think it is quite possible that MRSA and other resistant infections are not due to the misuse of antibiotics in our hospitals, but to the misuse of antibiotics given prophylactically in the meat industry.

Second, as we age and as we change our diet to include more processed foods, the amount of vitamin B12 we absorb may decline. For effective absorption of B12, it is necessary to have adequate saliva, stomach acid and pancreatic juices to detach the B12 from its initial protein, reattach it to the *intrinsic factor* in the stomach, absorb it in the small intestine and finally attach it

> **Def:** The *intrinsic factor* is an unidentified enzyme-like substance secreted by the stomach, present in the gastric juice and in the gastric mucous membrane.

to another protein so that it can be transported to the tissue. Any deficiency in the production of these digestive enzymes will decrease the amount of B12 absorbed, and these enzymes can be negatively affected by age, diet, toxins and medications. For example, the H2 and proton-pump inhibitors prescribed for gastric reflux, or metformin for diabetes, will diminish the absorption of B12.

The third cause of B12 deficiency is strictly technical – but it's important. The body uses the metabolically active forms of the vitamin, *methylcobalamin* and *adenosylcobalamin*, but the commercially available version of vitamin B12 available in drug stores is *cyanocobalamin*. This synthetic form of B12 is poorly absorbed, and must be metabolized by the liver into the two active forms of vitamin B12.

> ✧ ✧ ✧ ✧ ✧
> A deficiency of B12 becomes apparent first in the neurologic system.

It is preferable to use methylcobalamin when attempting to correct neurologic problems because of its affinity for the nervous system, but it can only be purchased at a compounding pharmacy. Methylcobalamin gets past the *blood-brain barrier* much more easily than cyanocobalamin. It is the more natural form of B12, more easily assimilated by the cells, and more readily utilized by the nervous system to correct a deficiency.

> ✧ ✧ ✧ ✧ ✧
> Note: See a full discussion of the *blood-brain barrier* in the next section.

Yet another cause of vitamin B12 deficiency is the tendency of toxins and heavy metals (such as mercury) to negatively affect the absorption of B12 and its eventual passage through the blood-brain barrier. When toxins are present in the *endothelial* cells, the great oxidative stress they create makes it more difficult for the B12 to get into the nervous system. That is why a patient's levels of serum B12 often do not accurately reflect the levels of B12 in the spinal fluid and nerve cells. Even though the

> **Def:** The *endothelium* is the thin layer of cells that lines the inside surfaces of our blood vessels. These specialized cells line the entire circulatory system, from the heart to the tiniest of our capillaries.

serum levels may seem adequate, they may be wholly inadequate to support the process of repairing the nervous system since the vitamin is prevented from getting past the blood-brain barrier.

Vegetarians, especially vegans, often have vitamin B12 deficiencies and need to take supplements, since B12 is obtained only through red meats and dairy products. The small amounts of B12 which may be artificially introduced into other foods such as cereals and milk are insufficient.

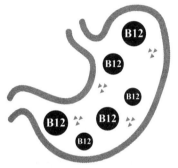

B12 remains trapped in protein if stomach acid is inadequate.

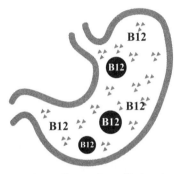

When there is sufficient stomach acid, B12 is released from protein.

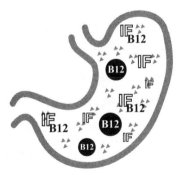

Intrinsic factor is needed before B12 can be used by your body.

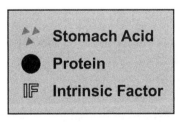

▲▲▲ **Stomach Acid**

● **Protein**

IF **Intrinsic Factor**

THE BLOOD-BRAIN BARRIER

The blood-brain barrier is often defined in medical textbooks as the mechanism by which the body prevents toxins and poisons from entering the brain. It consists of closely connected endothelial cells which line the capillaries in the brain, allowing only small molecules of glucose, small amino acids and gases (oxygen and carbon dioxide) to pass through, protecting the brain from all larger molecules including toxins.

> ❖ ❖ ❖ ❖ ❖
>
> The blood-brain barrier is a mechanism by which the body prevents toxins and poisons from entering the brain.

This sensitive arrangement can be compromised by many outside forces such as infection, inflammation, radiation, microwaves and even ultrasound. This is why it is probably wise to avoid heavy use of cell phones, since the microwave radiation they emit penetrates your head to a depth of about one inch.

The nervous tissue is also affected by excitotoxins, those small amino acid groups found in the food additive MSG and in aspartate molecules in sugar substitutes like Equal and NutraSweet.

These naturally occurring or synthetic chemicals found in very small amounts in our food over-stimulate our nerve cells, causing excitation to the point that they may fatigue and die. This excitation can also create misdirection and redirection of nerve synapses and pathways, creating aberrant behavior and neurophysiologic changes in our bodies that are detrimental to our general well being – and can trigger trigeminal neuralgia attacks. I highly recommend that TN patients carefully read food labels and avoid all excitotoxins and all products that have the words "partially hydrogenated vegetable oil" or "vegetable proteins" on their labels, since these imply that the foods could contain excitotoxins as well as trans-fats.

CHAPTER 15

VITAMIN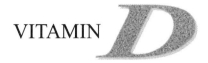

We've previously seen how certain micronutrient deficiencies can exacerbate trigeminal neuralgia and related facial pain. Examples of these are vitamin B12 and the essential fatty acids found in the omega 3s and omega 6s, which can be depleted through our choice of diet, exposure to environmental toxins and the effects of aging. However, there are other important micronutrients that are not related to these processes. Vitamin D is one of these.

Hydroxycalciferol, commonly called "vitamin D," is not a true vitamin but a pro-hormone, meaning it is the precursor to many of the hormones in our body including cholesterol, estrogen, testosterone and many other compounds.

Until recently, vitamin D was thought only to be involved in healthy bone production and maintenance. However, more recent research has shown it to be necessary for balance, for muscle and tendon health, to strengthen immunity and prevent infection, heart disease, cancer, autoimmune diseases and multiple sclerosis. The significant connection between a lack of vitamin D and multiple sclerosis suggests the intriguing possibility of using vitamin D in treating trigeminal neuralgia, since the pathology and the microscopic changes brought about by TN and multiple sclerosis are so similar and the illnesses are often confused.

> ❖ ❖ ❖ ❖ ❖
> Vitamin D is not a true vitamin but a pro-hormone.

Most foods – with the exception of fatty fish – are poor sources of vitamin D. Fortified foods such as milk, soy products and cereal grains are enriched with synthetic vitamin D2, which has to be metabolized in our bodies to create the active form of the vitamin. Each quart of milk is fortified with only about 100 international units of vitamin D, so meeting the daily requirements from food intake alone is a virtual impossibility.

Most vitamin D comes from the action of sunlight on cholesterol in the skin. The ultraviolet B rays from sunlight penetrate the skin, converting the cholesterol to a prohormone, which is then transformed into the active form of vitamin D. The amount of vitamin D formed in the skin depends on the skin pigmentation, age and health of the individual, plus the latitude of that individual's exposure to the sun. It may also depend upon the amount of cholesterol in the skin that is available to process.

> ❖ ❖ ❖ ❖ ❖
> Most vitamin D comes from the action of sunlight on cholesterol in the skin.

In most regions of the upper half of the United States during the winter months, it's highly unlikely that people will get enough sunlight to create an adequate amount of vitamin D. Research at the Massachusetts General Hospital showed that 57% of the patients coming through the emergency room during the winter have vitamin D insufficiency. Dark-skinned individuals especially suffer from lack of vitamin D since they have a natural "sunscreen" (melanin) that slows down the production of this vitamin.

A recent study in the *American Journal of Pediatrics* has shown that up to 42% of the African American teenagers may be deficient in Vitamin D due to dark pigmentation, diet and the latitude in which they live. Another significant factor affecting this issue is the increasing use of sunscreen and clothing worn to prevent skin cancer. While these recommendations are advocated by physicians, there is some evidence that skin cancer may be related to Vitamin D deficiency rather than ultraviolet exposure – and that there is little correlation between the deadly form of skin cancer (melanoma) and sun exposure.

The importance of Vitamin D to our overall health is underscored when we realize that fully 10% of our genes have Vitamin D receptors present on them. This is one micronutrient we want to be certain to keep fully supplied in our bodies!

Deficiency of vitamin D has been associated with cancer of the colon, prostate, breast and skin. It has been linked to tuberculosis, obesity, depression, schizophrenia, seasonal affective disorder, hypertension, cardiovascular disease and several autoimmune diseases including multiple sclerosis.

Research in the animal laboratory has shown that vitamin D is necessary for maintaining balance by regulating calcium flecks, or microliths, in the inner ear. This versatile vitamin is also necessary for muscle and tendon strength and is useful in reducing sports injuries. Vitamin D is stored in fat cells, so obese patients require a higher daily intake and have lower serum levels.

> ❖ ❖ ❖ ❖ ❖
> Vitamin D deficiency has been associated with cancer of the colon, prostate, breast and skin. It has been linked to tuberculosis, obesity, depression, schizophrenia, seasonal affective disorder, hypertension, cardiovascular disease and several autoimmune diseases including multiple sclerosis.

RECOMMENDED DOSAGES

Since optimizing vitamin D levels may be beneficial in so many ways, it is advisable to determine a vitamin D level in patients who have – or are susceptible to – the previously mentioned illnesses, and to implement the necessary supplementation.

The old recommended dose of 400 international units per day has now been increased to between 1,000 to 2,000 IU, depending on latitude and season, and on the pigmentation, age and general health of an individual. It's likely that 10,000 IU could be safely taken daily in most circumstances, as there have been no vitamin D toxicities reported under 10,000 IU per day. 50,000 IU a day has been given over a short term to patients with serious infections. Although toxicity is rare, high-dose vitamin D supplementation should only be used following consultation with your physician. Baseline blood levels of Vitamin D3 should be measured, and subsequent monitoring of these levels is recommended.

DRUG INTERACTIONS

Certain drug interactions will cause impairment to vitamin D absorption, such as protonics mineral oil, laxatives, obesity management medication (Orlistat), and bile acid sequestrants (Cholestyramine and Colestipol). Also, fat substitutes such as Olestra may decrease vitamin D absorption.

The symptoms of Vitamin D deficiency are many and varied, ranging from depression to bone pain. Medical professionals and educated patients (such as you are rapidly becoming) should always consider this possibility where the circumstances fit.

VITAMIN D AND CANCER

In 2005, a study demonstrated a beneficial correlation between vitamin D and prevention of cancer. This analysis of 63 published reports showed that taking an additional 1,000 IU of vitamin D daily reduced the risk of colon cancer by 50%, and breast and ovarian cancer by 30%. Further research has shown beneficial effects from high levels of vitamin D3 in patients with advanced prostate cancer. In a four-year clinical trial, vitamin D supplementation of 1,100 IU daily in a randomized intervention following 1,200 women reduced cancer incidence by 60%. If the cancers that originated in the first year were excluded (which were likely to have been present prior to intervention), the cancer reduction soared to 77%.

In 2007, the Canadian Cancer Society recommended that all young Canadian adults take 1,000 IU of Vitamin D during the fall and winter months. Research also suggests that cancer patients who have surgery done during the sunny summer have a better survival rate than patients whose surgeries are performed during the winter months. Data from four million cancer patients in 13 countries showed a marked difference in cancer rates between countries classified as sunny and countries classified as less sunny – and this was true for several different types of cancers.

VITAMIN D AND THE FLU

Dr. John J. Cannell, a psychiatrist from San Francisco, treated patients in his ward with high doses of vitamin D during a particularly virulent flu epidemic in 2005. More than 10% of the patients in the 1,200 bed hospital where he worked were infected by the virus, but none of the patients or staff in the ward that Dr. Cannell supervised contracted the disease. This observation was reinforced by an article in the *FASEB* Journal in 2005 by Adrian F. Gombart of the University of California at Los Angeles. He reported that vitamin D boosted the production of white blood cells in one of the antimicrobial compounds that defends the body against germs. This compound, called cathelicidin, targets microbes that include bacteria, viruses and fungal infections, as reported in the December 2008 issue of *Epidemiology and Infection*. The study noted the relationship between vitamin D and susceptibility to tuberculosis, which is an extremely difficult infection to prevent or control. Scientists stress the importance of supplementing with vitamin D3, which is the natural and active form of vitamin D, rather than with the synthetic vitamin D2 used in fortifying foods.

CHAPTER 16

Controlling Cholesterol

If I could take you into the operating room with me and show you the deposits of cholesterol on the arterial walls of a patient's heart – cholesterol deposited there by LDL when there was not enough HDL to carry it back through the lymph system and on to the liver where it could have been metabolized

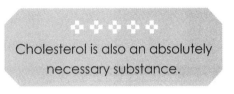

Cholesterol is also an absolutely necessary substance.

– you'd swear off butter, meat, ice cream and chocolate fudge sauce in a New York minute.

We hear about cholesterol primarily in relation to heart disease, and it is indeed one of the major causes – although *only* one – of that potential killer. But trigeminal neuralgia and related facial pain can also be affected by high cholesterol levels. Clearly, it can be a dangerous substance that TN patients must be aware of and understand well.

Cholesterol is also an absolutely necessary substance. It is an essential building block for our cells. When manufactured in the liver (someone once called the liver our "metabolic hotel"), it is carried by the bloodstream and deposited wherever cells need regeneration. So it's a fine balance between having too much or not enough cholesterol. But the important thing to remember is that it is the *quality* of the cholesterol – whether it's oxidized, whether it's HDL or LDL and even what size the LDL is – that counts. Oxidized cholesterol leads to increased inflammation and that can lead to a TN flare-up.

Cholesterol, a *lipid* compound, is also an essential component in the structure of nerve sheaths (TN patients take note) as well as cell membranes. Cholesterol is necessary for the production of hormones like estrogen, testosterone and vitamin D. The liver needs it to make bile. But once cholesterol enters into the wall of an artery and becomes oxidized, it attracts white cells and tissue-growth stimulators into the area of the vessel lining, leading to potentially life-threatening arterial blockages.

Def: *Lipids*: A broad group of naturally occurring molecules which includes fats, waxes, fat-soluble vitamins (A, D, E and K) and others.

Pernicious cholesterol is oxidized cholesterol. It enters our system by way of the foods we eat, particularly animal fats and dairy products. Even normal tissue conditions in the body can oxidize cholesterol. And even though our bodies make about 80 percent of our cholesterol, its production is stimulated by the fats we eat throughout our lives. Some of us can tolerate excess amounts of it far better than others, but it's bad for everyone.

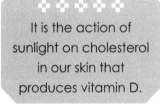

It is the action of sunlight on cholesterol in our skin that produces vitamin D.

We've seen that antioxidants prevent oxidation of cholesterol. They are vital, too, for the production, maintenance, and rejuvenation of our enzyme system, and they support and assist one another in eliminating the oxidative stress that can lead to harmful free-radical production. Some water-soluble antioxidants are vitamin C, albumen, thiol, and bilirubin. Fat-soluble antioxidants are vital in the management of cholesterol; examples include vitamins E, A and ubiquinone, also called Co-enzyme Q10 – CoQ10 for short.

Oxidation can be caused by perfectly normal cellular respiration, but also by infection, extreme exercise, physical and mental stress, inflammation – and by the foods we eat, such as saturated fats and trans-fats. The problem with refined and processed foods is that most of the antioxidants found in them in their natural state are destroyed during processing. Processed canned foods are usually high in sodium, which replaces magnesium and potassium – themselves antioxidants – in processing. When we eat refined flour, as found in bagels or white bread, we miss the benefits of the vitamin E found in unprocessed flour, which disappears from the wheat during processing. Then there are no antioxidants left to counter the stress that the flour itself imposes on our bodies.

Let's take a look at how cholesterol actually works in our bodies.

Picture yourself driving down the highway. You see a truck in the slow lane delivering cement to an area of the road under repair. Nothing to worry about. You continue driving, your progress unimpeded. But if a hundred cement trucks suddenly unloaded their cargo all at once, the cement would flow all over, spill onto the road, and slow your progress–even bring you to a halt.

As with cement, so it is with cholesterol. It is needed for "road repair." Under normal circumstances, the amount that's left over is cleared out by the body. But if an excess of cholesterol appears in the bloodstream – if there's more than the tissue needs or that the lymphatics can transport – then the excess piles up along the arterial walls, where it can cause reactions that will lead to hardening of the arteries.

As we've noted, two types of lipoproteins, the "good" high-density lipoprotein (HDL) and the "bad" low-density lipoprotein (LDL) are the important players here. LDL is a large, lightweight, fluffy molecule, much like a microscopic piece of popcorn; HDL is small and smooth, much like a miniature sunflower seed. That difference in shape is important: HDL is small and pliable enough to pass through the elastic membrane between the inner layer of the artery wall and into the lymphatic system in the outer layer. But LDL is too large to pass through the membrane. It is instead broken down into its components in the inner layer. Its amino acids pass through the membrane and are carried away by the lymphatics, but the debris that remains has to be dealt with. In adults, a ratio of 3.5 to 1.0, LDL to HDL, is considered healthy. But in some people, the ratio rises to 4.5 to 1, up to as much as over 8 to 1 – potentially disastrous levels.

❖ ❖ ❖ ❖ ❖
Cholesterol is essential for healthy nerve sheaths

If a large amount of HDL is present in the bloodstream and the arterial tissue, it will suck up the excess cholesterol and carry it through to the lymphatics, then into the venous system and into the liver for breakdown into bile acid, which is excreted through the small intestine. If the bile passes quickly through the intestines or is absorbed by waste material generated by a high-fiber diet, the cholesterol is eliminated. But if the bile stays in the system for too long, it is reabsorbed and converted back into cholesterol.

As I said, if excess cholesterol is not picked up by the HDL and carried to the liver, it still has to be dealt with by the body, because it's not good for it to just sit there. But here's the problem. Unfortunately, when cholesterol reaches the inner wall of the artery, it becomes oxidized – assuming it is not oxidized already – meaning that it carries an unpaired electron. That electron needs a mate, which it steals from a normal nearby molecule, thus destroying the healthy tissue components around it.

Oxidation renders the cholesterol very dangerous. Platelets and white cells stick to it. This is turn stimulates cell growth, leading to a potentially disastrous thickening of the arterial wall.

The white cells in the wall of the vessel recognize the oxidized cholesterol and ingest it, becoming *foam cells*. If no method is available for transporting the cholesterol, and if these foam cells become so full and aged that they rupture, the cholesterol is scattered into the lin-

> **Def:** *Foam cells* are microphages that have engulfed the oxidized cholesterol to prevent it from irritating nearby healthy tissue.

ing of the artery wall, setting up a tremendous inflammatory reaction. This is the beginning of arteriosclerotic plaque.

So cholesterol has been clearly implicated in the development of arteriosclerosis. Indeed, it may be the leading cause. If you have oxidized LDL and not enough HDL to carry it to your liver, an inflammatory reaction is sure to follow, causing arteriosclerosis.

> ❖ ❖ ❖ ❖ ❖
> I believe that TN, like arteriosclerosis, is a process of chronic inflammation.

This is also the case with trigeminal neuralgia: it is the inflammatory response that is so detrimental. I believe that TN, like arteriosclerosis, is a process of chronic inflammation caused by various agents working alone or together. Cholesterol is involved in all these processes because it is required in the repair of damaged tissues. It has been unfairly blamed as the cause of inflammation, when in some cases it is actually a key component in an attempt by the body to heal itself. It all depends on the balance between the amount of deposited oxidized cholesterol and the amount of HDL available to carry it away.

The incidence of arteriosclerosis is high in patients with elevated *C-reactive protein* levels. C-reactive protein is a marker for inflammation of many kinds and indicates higher risk regardless of a person's cholesterol levels. TN patients and those with arteriosclerosis also have elevated amounts of interleukin-1 (IL-1) and IL-6, proteins found in inflammatory illnesses.

Def: *C-reactive protein* (CRP) circulates in the bloodstream. Its levels rise and fall rapidly in response to inflammatory conditions in the body, making it a handy "marker" in identifying when an condition such as an infection exists, how advanced it is, and then how it is responding to treatment.

There is a correlation between chronic degenerative diseases, including TN and related nerve conditions, and certain other infectious processes: dental infections, viral infections, and infections involving the bacteria that cause stomach ulcers. Research is still going on in these areas, but I believe that in the near future medicine will recognize arteriosclerosis as a multifaceted process related to an inflammatory response to a variety of agents, which is the cause of the build-up in deposits of oxidized cholesterol. Prevention, therefore, should be directed toward removing or avoiding the cause of arteriosclerosis, and then limiting the inflammation. Oxidative stress, produced by the inflammatory process, can best be diminished by removing the irritants as quickly as possible.

GOOD FAT, BAD FAT

Although cholesterol can be considered a fat, not all fats contain cholesterol. Cholesterol is present only in the tissue of animals and in their milk products. Yet when you see a product that proclaims itself as "Cholesterol Free," you'll still find that it is often heavily made up of fat. Vegetable oils, for example, are 100% fat, but contain no cholesterol. Nevertheless, fat-laden foods like vegetable oil that have no cholesterol can still raise your cholesterol count.

The usefulness of fat is that it provides us with a fuel reserve. When you eat fat or sugar, your body's first reaction is to store it by making new cell membranes to enlarge the fat cells. To do this, your body makes extra cholesterol as an essential building block for manufacturing these cell walls, and for a variety of other purposes.

Current controversy rages over whether we should tolerate any added fat in our diet at all, because all additional dietary fats raise our level of cholesterol. This logic holds that even fish oil and vegetable oil can be harmful, so they should be cut out along with all animal fats. I think it's true that if we substitute fish oil and vegetable oil for the saturated fats found in meats, cream and cheese, we'll still have elevated cholesterol, simply because the American diet is so fat-heavy already – between 35 and 55 percent. If we simply substitute the same high amounts of vegetable and fish fat for all that saturated fat, we'll undoubtedly be better off, but we'll still be overweight and continue to have high cholesterol counts along with their attendant problems.

> ❖ ❖ ❖ ❖ ❖
> I firmly believe that 15 to 20 percent of our diet *should* be fat.

Should we cut out all added dietary fats? I don't think so. I firmly believe that 15 to 20 percent of our diet *should* be fat, provided this fat level is achieved by combining cold-pressed extra-virgin olive oil, fish oil, vegetable oil, essential fatty acids, and a very small amount of saturated fat – perhaps 1 or 2 percent. Certain vegetable oils like flaxseed oil (which is high in omega-3 fatty acids) and canola oil can be used in moderation for salads. Vegetable oils should not be used in cooking, because they oxidize easily when heated and can become very dangerous.

> ❖ ❖ ❖ ❖ ❖
> Vegetable oils should not be used in cooking, because they oxidize easily when heated.

The food industry processes polyunsaturated fats into saturated ones by breaking the extra chemical bonds and adding hydrogen – it's how they make margarine, for example, by converting a vegetable oil into a solid fat. Such processed polyunsaturated products can become trans-fats. These forms of fat are highly toxic. They decrease the production of vitamins, stimulate and oxidize cholesterol, and create oxidative stress. Antioxidants such as vitamins A and E occur naturally in vegetable oils, but when these polyunsaturated fats are processed, the antioxidants are removed. It's dangerous to ingest large amounts of processed vegetable oils to which no antioxidants have been added. For patients with facial neuralgias and other degenerative illnesses, such foods may create even more damage than saturated fats.

I want to reemphasize this point: *any* fats, whether or not manipulated polyunsaturated fats, when eaten in the large amounts that the American diet currently contains, will cause cholesterol problems. And those problems will surely contribute to the onset of many chronic diseases.

FISH AND FLAXSEED, NOT CHICKEN AND BEEF

Two fatty acids are essential for plasma cell membranes, for certain hormones, and for the regulation of the "messengers" that travel back and forth to activate or deactivate specific cells. These fatty acids are called omega-6 and omega-3. Omega-3 acids are found in many kinds of fish, such as tuna and salmon, in flaxseed oil, and in walnut oil – foods Americans should eat, but generally don't. Instead, we eat beef – thinking that if we cut off the fat, we'll be "watching our cholesterol" – and chicken, believing that it is lower in cholesterol than red meat.

In fact, though, both chicken and beef are destructive foods when eaten in large amounts. I eat no beef and almost no chicken; Janie eats neither. But I certainly understand the desire for these foods, and an occasional small portion most likely won't harm you. Removing a chicken's skin, along with its attendant fat, doesn't lower the amount of cholesterol you'll ingest, though it will definitely lower the amount of fat. The same holds true for beef; if you cut the fat off a steak, you'll lower your fat intake. But equal portions of this beef and the white meat of a chicken will contain about the same amounts of cholesterol.

The optimum level for cholesterol is different for every individual, and it makes no sense to look at these levels in a vacuum. Remember, it is oxidized cholesterol that's harmful, not cholesterol in general. Still, as an overall rule, the less cholesterol you eat, the healthier you'll be. "Good" cholesterol – the high-density lipoproteins (HDL) used as unoxidized building blocks for constructing your cell walls – is for the most part manufactured by your own body, and you'll easily get enough additional in your food to supplement it as needed. But the "bad" low-density lipoproteins (LDL) must be controlled, and that's up to you.

> ❖ ❖ ❖ ❖ ❖
> It is oxidized cholesterol that's harmful, not cholesterol in general.

Following the diet I have detailed in Chapter 10 will keep your overall cholesterol level down and build up the "good" HDL at the expense of the "bad" LDL. It is by far the best program I can recommend. Still, you may be tempted to take some shortcuts – cholesterol-lowering drugs, cholesterol-free and fat-free foods – and I want you to be aware of some facts before you make these important decisions.

COCONUT OIL

We have substituted coconut oil for many of the cooking oils in the recipes in Chapter 10 because new information has come to light to show the benefits of coconut oil in the human diet.

Coconut oil is used in many parts of the tropical world as a primary source of fat in diets. Millions of people also use it in cooking since it is very heat-stable, making it excellent for cooking and frying. Since coconut oil is so stable, it is slow to oxidize at high temperatures and resists rancidity. The high fatty acid content of coconut oil consists of about 50% lauric acid and 20% saturated myristic acid. Both of these are so-called "saturated acids" chemically "mid-carbon-chain" in molecular structure, meaning they have different effects on human health as opposed to the saturated fats that come from meats and artificially hydrogenated fats, both more common in our diets.

Coconut oil is 92% saturated fatty acids, 6% monounsaturated acids and 1.6% polyunsaturated acids. Careless processing of coconut oil can cause it to become partially hydrogenated, making it more solid with a higher melting temperature. Lauric acid is often separated out during processing due to its high value for medical applications. Coconut oil has been used in Asian curries and other Pacific-rim diets and relative to other cooking oils creates minimal harmful byproducts when heated. The calorie count of coconut oil is almost the same as other dietary fats Coconut oil has been used in studies which have shown a decrease in pneumonia in children at the Philippine Children's Medical Center where it was shown to accelerate the normalization of respiratory rate and resolution of pneumonia. A double-blind clinical trial with women to decrease obesity and promote reduction of obesity without causing abnormal lipid changes.

Coconut oil offers some wonderful health benefits, and it's a functional food. Research has shown that replacing other cooking oils in the diet with virgin coconut oil contributes to a more favorable HDL to LDL ratio. The oil is also antibacterial, antimicrobial and antiviral – and it contains several important nutrients. It has the greatest amount of saturated medium-chain triglycerides (62%) of any naturally occurring vegan food source for the more the lauric acid content (which approaches 50%) is significantly important in the immune system. The only other source of lauric acid found in such high concentrations is in mothers' milk. All other vegetable oils are completely devoid of these medium-chain fatty acids, which increase metabolism and make foods more easily digestible. They are processed directly in the liver and converted to energy therefore there is less strain on the digestive system. Research has also shown that coconut oil can improve cholesterol and lower blood pressure, and help with cardiac problems and infections. Coconut oil has been helpful in many other ways, including dental disease, osteoporosis, pancreatitis, kidney and liver disease.

BEWARE OF "FAT-FREE" FOODS

Yesterday, I went to my local supermarket to check out fat-free cookies, fat-free cakes, fat-free yogurt, and fat-free ice cream as options in my meals today. For breakfast, I could have made apple-cinnamon muffins from a fat-free mix (0 cholesterol, 130 calories per muffin). For lunch, I might have had a portion of fat-free raspberry chunk marble ice cream (0 cholesterol, 110 calories per serving) or fat-free frozen vanilla yogurt (0 cholesterol, 70 calories) for dessert, perhaps garnished with a fat-free devils food cookie (0 cholesterol, 50 calories). For dessert after dinner, I could have eaten a nice slab of angel food cake (0 cholesterol, 140 calories) topped by a scoop of fat-free chocolate ice cream (0 cholesterol, 90 calories) covered with fat-free real chocolate-flavored syrup (0 cholesterol, 110 calories).

But I didn't buy any of them. Instead, I settled for some melon at breakfast, a mix of blueberries and strawberries after lunch, and no dessert at dinner – just green tea. I don't trust fat-free foods. There are less risky alternatives out there.

Despite our national obsession with fat-free foods, few consumers take the time to investigate what they are really eating – what, if any, nutritional benefits they are deriving, and whether they might be better off avoiding cookies, cakes, frozen yogurt and ice cream altogether. Rather, they see the proclamation "Fat-Free!" or "Reduced Fat" on the labels and they eat these products with a feeling of virtue. They then proceed to eat the rest of their normal diet, heavy with meat and poultry, thinking that at least they've cut down on fatty foods and given themselves a nutritional boost.

> ❖ ❖ ❖ ❖ ❖
> I don't trust fat-free foods. There are less risky alternatives out there.

Of course, if people *did* take the time to investigate, they'd soon be mired in confusion. They'd find that some cookies contain little fat and no cholesterol, while a 1/2 cup serving of chocolate chip cookie-dough premium ice cream contains 14 grams of fat and a whopping 65 mg of cholesterol – one-third of an entire day's sensible total amount – to say nothing of 270 calories per serving. They'd also find that some virtually fat-free foods (shrimp, for example) are very high in cholesterol. And some products whose labels proudly proclaim them to be "Fat Free!" (such as cereals and some crackers) shouldn't contain any fat because they're made from grain. People would be much better off worrying about the amount of sugar these foods contain, because sugar turns into fat once it's in the body.

I suppose the best thing I can say about fat-free foods is that they're better for you than fat-rich foods. Still, we go on eating foods that are high in fat, such as cheese, meat and poultry, thinking that by cutting down on other "fatty" foods like cake and ice cream, we've done enough in the way of dietary self-control. Then doubt creeps in. Our weight remains constant, or goes up. Unlovable "love handles" appear above our hips. And even worse, our cholesterol level also rises. Four years ago it was at 190. Two years ago it rose to 210, not yet alarming, but cause for concern. Now it's up to 240, and our internist lectures us: "Too high," she says. "You're putting yourself in harm's way. Better lower your cholesterol, and lower it *now* or you're in trouble." She writes out a diet of mostly vegetables and fruits, perhaps prescribes a formidable vitamin and supplement regimen that entails taking more than twenty pills a day, and tells us to come back in a year – no more of those two-year breaks between checkups.

But what about those business lunches and dinners, the cocktail parties and the afternoon teas featuring Muriel's "all-butter" lemon loaf? What about the celebrations, holidays and family get-togethers? Just because *our* cholesterol is high doesn't mean we should deny our friends and family the foods they love, does it? And of course, just to be sociable, we might join them at the table, just this once....

We can't seem to change our diet radically enough, and on too many of these social occasions, our will power simply fails. So our cholesterol levels continue to rise, and now we're in real trouble. We begin to think that the only solution is to try one of those cholesterol-lowering drugs. After all, aren't they supposed to be almost magical?

DO DRUGS HELP LOWER CHOLESTEROL?

Let's agree on a few basic facts.

❖ It is clear that high blood-cholesterol levels are associated with coronary artery disease. It is not the *only* cause – there are many instances when arteriosclerosis is not associated with cholesterol at all – but it is *a* cause, and it would be foolish not to try to minimize that risk.

❖ It is also clear that when you lower your cholesterol level, you lower your risk of heart attack. Lower your cholesterol by 2 points and your risk of heart attack drops by 1 percent. Lower it by 20 points and your risk drops by 10 percent – a meaningful improvement.

❖ It is not a question of *whether* you should lower your cholesterol level, it is only a question of *how*.

Ideally, we would change our diets, increase our exercise, and re-center ourselves to respond healthfully to stress. But as we've seen, some people don't have the will, the time, or the inclination. They look to drugs to do the work for them.

❖ ❖ ❖ ❖ ❖
Cholesterol-lowering drugs should never be used as a substitute for maintaining a low-cholesterol, low-fat diet.

Cholesterol-lowering drugs can stop the progression of arterial plaque formation, and in some cases they can actually cause a reduction of the existing built-up plaque. They are especially helpful in limiting "soft plaques," reducing the chances of bits of plaque splitting off and causing an obstruction by clot formation. But there are side effects, particularly if the drugs are used as an excuse for continuing to eat a high-fat diet. Remember that cholesterol-lowering drugs should never be used as a substitute for maintaining a low-cholesterol, low-fat diet. In fact, taking them as an antidote to high-fat meals actually exposes the patient to the most serious side effects of these drugs.

Still, I do prescribe them from time to time, often with substantial benefits to my patients. They're most effective in young people with a high LDL-to-HDL ratio who have not been able to lower their cholesterol without drugs. If a six-week "natural" regimen doesn't work, then I'll turn to drugs.

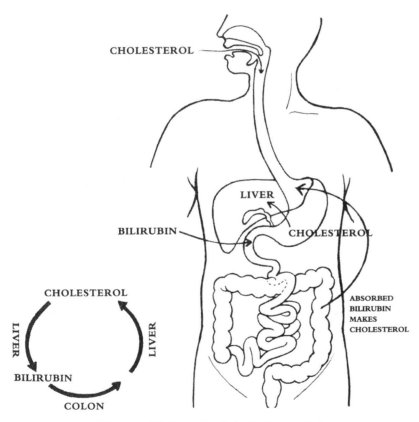

Diagram of cholesterol cycle in the human body

STATIN DRUGS

The statin drugs – simvastatin (Zocor), pravastatin (Pravachol), lovastatin (Mevacor), atorvastatin (Lipitor) – are perhaps the most effective, and the most dangerous, of the cholesterol-lowering drugs. They work by blocking one of the enzymes that create cholesterol.

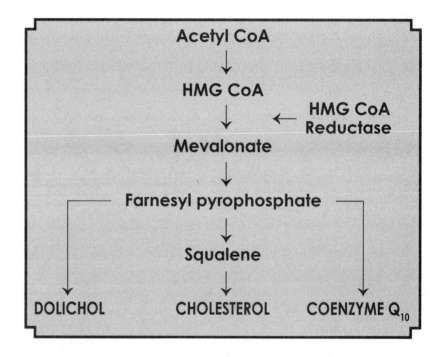

The problem is that they also block the production of other essential compounds, such as CoQ10 – both a powerful antioxidant and a bio-energy producer necessary for the cells to produce fuel important to bodily functions. People with trigeminal neuralgia need to be especially diligent in keeping up their levels of CoQ10 – mainly through supplements – for many reasons.

A shortage of CoQ10 can affect the immune system and even cause heart failure, among other disorders. Hypersensitivity reaction to statin drugs may also occur, leading to inflammation of the lung tissues, rashes, heart disease, fatigue, joint pain, psoriasis, shortness of breath, and swelling of feet and hands. Such symptoms occur in about 8 percent of patients who take statin drugs. Liver failure, gallbladder disease, and lupus-like symptoms have also been reported, along with more-common complaints of discomfort, gassiness, bloating and cramps. Early studies of statin drugs reported higher incidence of cancer (researchers at the University of San Francisco found that the statins are carcinogenic in other animals), suicide and mental instability. Some doctors have associated statin drugs with Alzheimer's disease because they can lower cholesterol levels beyond the point where enough remains to properly repair brain cells and their protective linings. This caution applies equally to TN patients. Lowering your cholesterol level too much may actually cause your trigeminal neuralgia symptoms to re-emerge, because not enough available cholesterol may lead to decay of the nerve sheaths – a prescription for big trouble for TN patients

Why, then, would anybody take statin drugs? – Because they are effective, and because it is possible to supplement them with micronutrients to prevent some of their side effects. Since taking statins depletes CoQ10, and because a patient would exhibit symptoms from this loss – such as muscle weakness, fatigue, and soreness – supplementing the statin drugs with CoQ10 has proved successful in many cases. If patients who have tried this combination still suffer a hypersensitivity reaction manifested by hives, rash or pneumonia, then statin drugs should be discontinued, since these symptoms are the result of taking the drug, not the additional CoQ10.

So by all means, be careful. The immensely profitable statin drugs have been loudly and widely advertised by the drug industry. It's hard to spend an evening in front of the tube without seeing an ad for Lipitor, but the possible harmful side effects – mentioned in a babbling low voice or shown in tiny print – are played down, when to my mind they should be strongly stressed. Miracle drugs statins may be, but risk-free they most assuredly are not.

CHAPTER 17

Aging

Aging is not a disease. Indeed, it can be a blessing. Yet in Western cultures – particularly in the U.S. – it is a condition to be avoided for as long as possible. We are constantly urged to fight against the "aging process." Television ads and sitcoms are targeted mainly toward attracting young viewers, and we seem to have the mindset that being "30-something" is already a long way toward the grave. Aging to us, as Stephan Rechtschaffen[12] writes, is "an anathema. It's as though every new wrinkle requires a smoothing cream, every grey hair a dye, every aching joint a liniment. We run from aging, we deny it, and we are embarrassed by it."

In other societies, especially in Asian ones, old age is known as a time of wisdom, of tranquility, of contemplation and spirituality. The elderly are honored, not ignored. They are consulted and listened to, admired and seen as reliable purveyors of knowledge gained through long personal experience. Such knowledge is less about facts and more about the emotional and instinctual sides of our being. They've "been there; done that," and they can teach us life's lessons if we will just be patient and listen.

---

[12] Stephan Rechtschaffen is co-founder of the Omega Institute for Holistic Studies and author of the book Timeshifting.

THE BIOLOGY OF AGING

No one beyond the age of about 21 really *wants* to get any older, but of course we all do want to live as long as possible. We know that the process of living has both qualitative and quantitative aspects, but even if the quality of our life is poor, physically or emotionally, we usually want to prolong it. As the old saying goes, "it's better than the alternative." We want to live into old age healthily and productively, avoiding deterioration as much as possible along the way. We want to maintain physical agility and mental acuity, to be – as the mother of a friend of mine is – "a young 95."

The scientific community has long studied the aging process intensely. Aging questions are many: Why do cells stop multiplying (although we now know that brain cells do regenerate late into life)? Why do bones become brittle? Why does hair grey? Why does memory fail? These questions and others have been studied extensively, and in the past few decades, much new evidence has come to light. In the 1970s, research first pointed to free radicals and oxidative stress as the cause not only of many chronic degenerative diseases, but of aging itself. Since then, further study of aging has validated the theory that oxidation of lipids and the mutation and breakdown of DNA are important components of the aging process.

A continuing mystery of aging is *apoptosis* – programmed cell death, in which a cell's function winds down so that eventually it fails to metabolize and simply dies. Microscopic examination of an apoptotic cell shows an essentially normal-looking cell that has one dramatic drawback: it no longer functions. Current theory holds that at some point the DNA in the cell sends it a message that it is time to shut down its metabolic energy plant and stop reproducing – in effect, programming its own death. This process can be greatly accelerated by the forces of oxidative stress, even though it is inevitable over time.

Another important factor in the aging process is *glycation*[13], the caramelizing or burning of the *glycoproteins* in our bodies. When oxidative stress occurs, it attacks the sugar in the glycoprotein, which caramelizes in much the same way sugar heated in a saucepan becomes light brown as it oxidizes. The trouble here is that when glycation takes place, the glycoprotein loses its integrity and becomes useless in hormonal reactions, a common condition in aging adults that leads to lower levels of all kinds of hormones.[14]

> **Def:** *Glycoproteins* are chemical compounds made of sugar and protein that are an integral part of our tissue.

This stress-related biology lesson (weren't all biology lessons stressful in school?) ends with the body's production of *metalloprotease*, the enzymes that break down the proteins in *collagen* and *elastin*. These enzymes are released in inflammatory reactions or under oxidative stress, resulting in the breaking of the collagen bonds and the elastic membrane layer that maintain the integrity of various tissues including arteries and skin, resulting in sagging and wrinkles.

---

[13] Sugar is added to many processed food products primarily to enhance browning and improve appearance, rather than to add sweetness. A partial list: French fries, barbecued meats, dark-colored cola drinks and many baked goods - doughnuts and cakes among them.

In products where high cooking temperatures are involved, sugars combine with proteins or fats to create dangerous chemical compounds. There is good evidence that these types of processed foods contribute to a range of age-related degenerative diseases, from retinal dysfunction and type II diabetes to cardiovascular disease. Just one more reason to avoid processed foods in your diet.

[14] Age spots – those brown spots on the skin – are clear visible examples of this "human caramelizing"

The unifying factor in all these processes in oxidative stress, which is why I say that if you make an effort to minimize it, you can effectively slow the aging process itself. Besides the standard principals for antioxidation we've described in this book, slowing the effects of aging can be enhanced with the Lemole formula of decreasing your body's toxic load, reinforcing the antioxidative defenses, and improving the lymphatic flow to clear your body of toxins and inflammatory by-products. Along with the antioxidants included in my 14-Day Diet, I'd add 500 mg of alpha lipoic acid three times daily to help prevent DNA mutation and migration of inflammatory messengers. Other useful supplements to slow the aging process are para-aminobenzoic acid (PABA) to preserve skin elasticity, and pantothene to promote healthy hair and lessen graying and baldness.

OTHER AGING PROBLEMS AND TREATMENTS

Bone shrinkage is a sign of aging. It not only causes osteoporosis and spine deformity, but also changes the appearance of the face. Jaw and cheekbones recede, causing facial tissue to sag and teeth to loosen in their sockets. Exercise will slow bone shrinkage by increasing cardiovascular and muscle tone, and will normalize bone architecture by preserving calcium and magnesium.

Another challenge is loss of water in the skin. Salves and creams help this condition, as does living in a less-than-bone-dry atmosphere. Limit your direct sun exposure to minimize drying and protect against both wrinkles and skin cancer. That sour look that sometimes develops with old age probably has less to do with bitterness and more to do with magnesium deficiency; an additional 400 to 1,200 mg per day will give a glow to your face. And if you want to avoid those dark rings under your eyes that can come with advancing age, cut back or give up alcohol and coffee.

Smoking, along with its many other deadly consequences, causes artery spasms in the skin which destroy the small muscles beneath the surface, which in turn lead to the formation of scar tissue under the skin's surface – the cause of wrinkles. I've often thought the best way to stop girls and young women from smoking is to forget about their cancer risks and instead threaten them with premature aging. Might as well bring out the big guns when you have them!

AGING "TREATMENTS"

- ✤ Eat a diet high in complex carbohydrates, including fresh vegetables and fruits and featuring monounsaturated and polyunsaturated oils.

- ✤ Avoid animal fats, coconut fats, trans-fats, hydrogenated oils and shortening.

- ✤ Include in your diet omega-3 fatty acids, including walnut oil, fish oil, and pumpkin, sunflower and sesame seeds.

- ✤ Add supplements to your diet: folic acid, vitamins A and E, essential fatty acids, lecithin, zinc, aloe vera and jojoba oil.

- ✤ Use a good skin moisturizer every day.

- ✤ Avoid over-exposure to direct sunlight and avoid tanning beds altogether. When you go out in the sun, wear a broad-brimmed hat and sunglasses.

- ✤ Use only mild soaps and cleaning products.

- ✤ Buy a humidifier for your home.

- Exercise regularly to increase blood and lymph circulation, and to build oxygen intake. The 95-year-old woman I mentioned walks a mile a day and uses light weights to maintain her upper-body strength.

- Begin a regular massage program.

- Practice relaxation techniques such as yoga or tai chi.

- Meditate.

- Maintain an optimistic outlook on life. A positive attitude offers real, quantifiable physical benefits, and makes life much happier for you and for those around you.

- Follow your choice of regular spiritual practice.

The regimen for aging is much like the one I recommend for all ages. It only stands to reason that if we avoid exposure to strong oxidative triggers, follow a sensible diet and adopt a solid exercise program, we can extend the functional age of our bodies and minds. The river of life can flow for many years in each of us. But we cannot take it for granted – it is entirely up to us to make sure it keeps flowing smoothly.

CHAPTER 18

Suicide and Violence

One of the more serious problems I've seen related to treating trigeminal neuralgia is an increased risk of suicide. Patients with long-standing, unrelenting pain and incapacitation can become severely depressed and entertain suicidal thoughts – or actually attempt the act. The cause of these symptoms is further confounded by the fact that many of the drugs used in treating trigeminal neuralgia have been associated with increased suicidal tendencies. Is it the pain, the depression or the drugs – or drug combinations? Or is it the complex relationship of all three of these components affecting a less-than-totally-resilient individual?

Dr. Susan Kobassa, a psychologist of City University of New York, defines resiliency as "the ability to recover from, or adjust to, change or misfortune." No one likes change, but it is inevitable. Mark Twain said, "The only person who likes change is a wet baby." So our coping skills and resiliency allow us to adjust positively to change and overcome misfortune.

Dr. Kobassa says that a resilient person exhibits 3 Cs:

1. *Commitment* to task;

2. Personal *control* recognition – to realize what can be controlled and what has to be accommodated to;

3. Challenge to be overcome rather than accepted fatalistically.

Fortunately, there are programs for resiliency training to help improve patients' attitudes in facing serious illness, depression or trauma.

Having said that, there remains a darker concern that anti-convulsant drugs, anti-depressants and SSRIs[15] can increase the tendency to suicide. That is why the use of any of these medications – especially in the early phase or during withdrawal – should be closely monitored by a physician. Subtle or casual thoughts or inclinations regarding suicide should be immediately reported to your doctor. Although the risk is quite small, it is also quite real.

The confounding combination of persistent pain, depression and drug effects makes it difficult to positively prove any relationship between the medication and a tendency toward suicide. However, several studies have been helpful in determining cause by looking at the drugs used in other diseases not associated with pain or depression (or taking into account depression). In 2004, the FDA issued a warning about the heightened risk of suicide in patients taking Wellbutrin as well as Prozac, Paxil, Zoloft, Effexor, Celexa, Remeron, Lexapro, Luvox and Serazone. Then in 2008, the FDA required that all drugs in the anticonvulsant class carry a warning that they double the risk of suicidal thoughts and behavior. As recently as April 2010, a research team from Harvard, headed by Dr. Elisabetta Patorno, found that patients on anticonvulsant medication such as Neurontin, Lamictal, Trileptil, Gabitril and Valproate had 2.5 times the incidence of suicidal attempts. This was a five-year

---

[15] Selective serotonin reuptake inhibitors are a group of compounds often prescribed as antidepressants. Along with some possible increase in suicidal thoughts, there are known SSRI interactions with several drugs commonly prescribed in TN treatment, including carbamazepine (Tegretol) and phenytoin (Dilantin).

study of 300,000 patients that showed, although small, the risk was quite real and recommended that "Both patients and health care professionals should be alert to early symptoms that might potentially be associated with suicidal risks." Dr. Patorno concluded, "Physicians should discuss associated risks and benefits with their patients, and *together* determine the best treatment course."

I've had experience with several patients who had no pain but were mildly depressed – and although they didn't have trigeminal neuralgia, their stories can alert us to the importance of not only proper medication, but also the appropriate dosage.

Gavan, a 60-year old caretaker and part time teaching assistant, lived with his mother and father and extended family. Eventually his parents died, and then he lost his job and developed epilepsy. He became somewhat depressed and was placed on Wellbutrin. In a short time he developed suicidal thoughts. He planned his suicide – and I mean he sat down and planned it as though he was cooking a casserole. Fortunately he realized this was abnormal since he had never before experienced these tendencies. He went to the hospital and asked to be admitted. He stayed there for three days before being discharged on a *higher* dose of Wellbutrin. His physician said the initial dose was inadequate and this had created the dangerous situation Gavan experienced. He has been functioning normally on the higher dose of medication.

Rob was a 74-year old Korean War Veteran on the GI Bill who I knew in college. "Big Bob" was a quiet, good guy – it took a lot to make him angry. After school, we got together a couple of times, but we lost touch when he moved to the South with his family.

A few years ago, a mutual friend asked me, "Did you hear about Bob? He murdered his wife! He's in jail for life." Knowing what a stand-up guy he was, I found it hard to believe. Through the Internet, I got the story from the local newspaper. Bob had claimed he wasn't guilty. The prosecutor said, to paraphrase, "Well, your wife was found dead in your house, and you were standing on the porch. The window was shot out and your gun was on the floor – with your fingerprints on it."

The evidence seemed very convincing.

I wrote Bob a letter telling him how sorry I was about his tragedy. He wrote back: "Thanks to Merck & Co. and Paxil, I'm in here for life." I didn't know what he was talking about and wrote again to ask him why he thought that. In his response, he directed me to a website that discusses more than 2,000 violent crimes committed by patients on SSRIs. I was astounded by the number of cases that were associated with the prescribed use of these drugs.[16]

Bob told me that he had a happy life with his wife, that he had loved her dearly and that there was no argument or any other reason for him to commit this violent crime. He had been placed on Paxil for mild depression not long before the crime, and he said he remembered nothing about the violence.

These are just two examples of the severe problems that may arise as a result of taking medications commonly used in controlling trigeminal neuralgia and related facial pain. The application of these powerful drugs must be carefully monitored – not only for the appropriateness of any given medication, but also for the correct dosage.

---

[16] If you'd like to review this subject in detail, go to: www.ssristories.com.

CHAPTER 19

Gwen's Story and Other Successes

Several years ago my sister-in-law, Gwen Asplundh, called Janie for help. She had been previously diagnosed with trigeminal neuralgia and consequently had run the gauntlet of conventional medicine – from drugs to the gamma-knife procedure.

But her symptoms always returned. Gwen asked Janie if there were any holistic remedies for her persistent disease. Janie went into the investigation full throttle, searching journals, papers, books and audio tapes. She developed a program, which I reviewed and Gwen then adopted. It seemed logical enough to me, and at least harmless. Lo and behold, after six weeks Gwen was pain free and has, for the most part, remained so ever since.

I hope other people suffering with incapacitating trigeminal neuralgia and related facial pain can be significantly helped through such a nutritional approach to health, along with the crucial balancing factors of effective stress management and appropriate exercise.

Gwen's journey through fear and pain – and her ultimate relief – is best described in her own words. It is an articulate and touching description of how her disease progressed, how her family supported her, and how she finally triumphed over TN.

An address given to the Trigeminal Neuralgia Association,
November 12, 2004.

This is a story of natural healing – a story of escaping daily reliance on drugs to control pain. My suffering will be very familiar to my fellow TN sufferers; this concerns the debilitating pain, the utter misery and hopelessness of TN patients. TN pain completely takes over your life, affecting you and your loved ones so that a normal life is impossible.

My first attack was in April, 1993 – a sharp pain in the lower jaw and teeth on the left side. Thinking it was an infected tooth and I probably needed root canal, I went to my dentist. After examination, he concluded that the pain was not tooth-related, but sent me to a root-canal specialist for a second opinion. I came very close to having a perfectly good tooth pulled; in fact the doctor had his gloves on, ready to operate, when I told him I still had pain even though he had anaesthetized the area. He took off his gloves, said there was probably nothing wrong with my tooth, and recommend I see a neurologist. Because the pain subsided shortly afterwards, I didn't do anything more at that time.

For the next two years I went through periods of pain and remission. The pain was never so bad during this time that I couldn't handle it. In February of 1995, the pain set in with a vengeance: sharp, excruciating pain in my left upper and lower jaws would come for a few minutes or longer, off and on, and then fade, leaving a strange burning sensation along my tongue on that side. Chewing food was out of the question, communicating was accomplished with written notes since speaking was too painful, and brushing my teeth became a thing of the past. I prayed I wouldn't sneeze. The pain lessened when I lay down, but every time I swallowed it hit again. I can remember trying to take as long as I possibly could between swallows. In my experience, no pain killers are effective against TN pain. But some nights I would take Percocet or Tylenol with codeine which at least made me drowsy so I could sleep.

My husband called Sue Remmey, the chairperson of our Philadelphia TN support group. She was wonderfully sympathetic and helpful, just the person we needed when we felt so desperate. Sue recommended we see a neurologist, which we did, and he started me on Tegretol. Following this we had a conference with Dr. Casey asking if we would consider having an MVD procedure. He felt that was too radical an approach so early in the game, and counseled me to continue with the Tegretol.

After a few months I became allergic to Tegretol, developing a rash. So my medication was changed to Neurontin. While I could tolerate Neurontin, it was not very successful in alleviating my pain. In April of 1996, the doctor decided to try Baclofen instead of the ineffective Neurontin. This definitely was not a good move for me! The side effects of Baclofen were bad news. My motor skills were severely affected. I kept dropping things. One night I fell when I got out of bed because my knee gave way. I couldn't make sense of what I was reading. I felt like crying all the time. I slept much more than normal. And to make matters worse – the pain not only didn't go away, it got worse! So back I went to Neurontin.

By now, I was beginning to feel that I needed to take some sort of radical step as I was obviously getting nowhere with the medications. So I decided to try stereotactic radiosurgery, or what is called gamma-knife. This procedure appealed to me because it didn't involve an incision into the brain.

In June, 1996, Dr. Kondziolka performed the gamma-knife procedure on me at University Presbyterian Hospital in

Pittsburgh. At first I was elated, as I had immediate relief, but five months later the pain returned. What a terrible disappointment! The pain was never as debilitating as before, but certainly it was bad enough that we couldn't live a normal life. I have heard many conflicting opinions on the success of the gamma-knife from doctors and patients alike. But from my experience, I wouldn't recommend it.

So there I was, back on the less-than-effective Neurontin, limping along. By now I had tried acupuncture, homeopathic remedies, massage, drug medication and gamma-knife. I was feeling pretty devastated.

Through all this, I was blessed with a truly loving, supportive family and friends. My husband and children couldn't have been more concerned or helpful. My husband was there for me through every crisis, doing his best to help in any and every way he could. He never complained about how my affliction was affecting his life, as indeed it was.

Next in my retinue of supporters are Emily Jane Lemole and her husband, Dr. Gerald Lemole. Janie is my husband's sister – our next-door neighbor and very dear friend. She is an omnivorous reader on all matters pertaining to health. She has taken graduate courses in nutrition and lectured on the subject. She is married to a busy cardiac surgeon. Her son-in-law also is a cardiac surgeon, and one of her sons is a neurosurgeon. Janie has many interests, including a large family, world-wide travel, and the tireless pursuit of personal growth and study. Janie brings a unique and inspiring perspective to the most important health issues of our times. She is always ready and willing to give herself to those in need, as is her husband. Together they are truly a wonderful team.

In the spring of 1997, Janie asked me if I wouldn't like to try a new approach to treating my pain. She had read about a successful treatment of TN patients using diet and supplements in a medical book titled *Putting it all Together: the NEW Orthomolecular Nutrition* by Abram Hoffer, M.D., Ph.D., & Morton Walker, D.P.M. Although I was skeptical, I decided I had nothing to lose.

Treatment begins with liquid Vitamin B12 by injection several times a week (I did it daily at first), tapering off as the pain lessens, and discontinuing when the pain goes away. Thereafter you continue with B12 in a sublingual form. We found that the injections were critical to the success of this program for me. At the same time as the injections, I took the vitamins that were recommended. I also followed a dairy- and sugar-free diet on Dr. Hoffer's recommendation.

After two to three weeks of this program, I felt I was part of a miracle. I was able to go off Neurontin, we could discontinue the B12 injections and I was pain-free! How wonderful to not have to depend on mind-numbing drugs for pain relief. Instead, I am eating a healthy diet, taking my vitamins and supplements, and thanking the Lord every day that I wake up without pain. In more than seven years, I have not had to take *any* drugs.

During this period I have had a few recurrences of pain brought on sometimes by stress, once by a severe bout of diarrhea which eliminated all the nutrients as fast as I took them, and twice by Lyme disease. When this happens, I have been able to bring the pain under control again by going back on the B12 injections as needed. I have also started various other treatments at these "pain breakout" times.

For obvious reasons, I am a firm believer in Orthomolecular Medicine which takes into account the nutritional needs of patients. This practice recognizes the individuality of each person and that some people require very large amounts of specific nutrients.

If you do decide to try this program, you may meet with resistance from your doctor (and of course we recommend that you do confer with her or him before making any changes in your treatment.) Your doctor may say that you don't need B12 injections – that oral products are just as effective. Or, if you do take injections, you don't need them often. You may be told that too much Vitamin C is excessive. Most medical doctors are not nutritionists and have not been educated in using natural healing. They are uncomfortable with these methods, which they feel have not been demonstrated by lengthy testing.

I highly recommend this all-natural program to anyone suffering with TN pain. I know it's hard to believe that a program that doesn't rely on drugs or surgical procedures can be effective. I also know that what works for one person may not work for another. But doesn't the reward of being without pain and off drugs make it worth giving the natural path a try? What have you got to lose?

FOLLOW-UP NOTE

Unfortunately, Gwen had a TN recurrence in 2010 that required a balloon dilation, followed by an additional mini-procedure, and she has responded well. But the variation of ortho-molecular therapy that Janie and I devised had kept her well and intervention free for 13 years.

FOUR OTHER SUCCESS STORIES

Gwen is not alone in her success. Here are four more testimonials – all involving patients of mine –describing the wonderful results patients have experienced from the Lemole Recovery Program:

RYAN

Ryan was 72 when he came to our office complaining of severe stabbing pain in his left cheek – so terrible that he had been unable to eat solid foods and had lost 35 pounds due to the condition. He had first suffered with this pain four years earlier. No diagnosis had been made at that time, and the pain had receded temporarily.

We treated Ryan with high doses of vitamin B12 intramuscularly every day. In less than one week, the pain was less frequent, less severe and not as "stabbing." Two months later, Ryan was still doing well.

KELLY

Kelly was a 54-year-old woman who came to us with feelings of burning in her head and intense, zap-like pains above her lip. She had suffered with this for years. She had sought treatment at several hospitals and from several dentists. She had even had teeth extracted, but nothing had helped her pain. Dr. Lemole diagnosed Kelly as most likely having trigeminal neuralgia. Treatment included high-dose vitamin B12 shots weekly. Over a period of time, the pain was reduced and finally disappeared completely. Kelly continued to take B12 shots for several more years.

NICOLE

Nicole was a 46-year-old secretary who had gone to a dentist for a root canal and had suffered severe pain during the examination. The pain started in her head and then traveled to her right ear and then to her jaw, stabbing and constantly "zapping" her. Sometimes her vision became blurry in her right eye.

An Ear, Nose and Throat doctor gave a diagnosis of tonsillitis or perhaps nerve damage from the root canal procedure. Nicole was given Neurontin 300 mg three times daily. This did not resolve the problem.

When Dr. Lemole examined Nicole, he diagnosed trigeminal neuralgia and discontinued the Neurontin. Nicole was placed on the Lemole trigeminal neuralgia recovery program, including vitamin B12 shots.

Within a few months, Nicole had regained her color and healthful appearance. Her TN pain took more than a year to fully resolve, but there was dramatic improvement in only a matter of months.

JESSICA

Jessica was a 42-year-old who had been diagnosed with trigeminal neuralgia 11 months before coming to see Dr. Lemole. Her symptoms were a burning pain in her right jaw, plus burning lips and tongue. Her face was sensitive even to very light touch. She had been taking Neurontin, 300 mg three times a day, together with vitamins C, E, and B12.

Dr. Lemole placed Jessica on the Lemole Recovery Program, including high-dose vitamin B12 shots.

After only 12 days, Jessica's pain was nearly gone, with only a few remaining occasional twitches. She continued with Neurontin 300 mg, decreased to only once a day, and vitamin B12 injections every three days.

USDA Food Pyramid, 70

Vegetable, 125
Vegetable and Rice, 125
    Broccoli Baobabs, 87, 126
    Christopher's Rice, 88, 126
    French Un-Fries, 84, 86, 128
    Stuffed Acorn Squash, 88, 127
Vegetables and Rice, 125
    Spanish Rice, 88, 125
Vegetable and Rice Dishes, 125
Vegetarian, 15, 23, 55, 72-74, 131, 219
    Fat-Free Seitan Steak Marsala, 131
    Seitan Pot Roast, 132
    Vegetarian Sausage and Zucchini
    Saute, 132
Vegetarian Cheese Steak Sandwiches,
    117
Vegetarian Diet Pyramid, (*illus.*).79
Vegetarian Entrees, 131
Vegetarian Sausage and Zucchini Saute,
    132
Vitamin C, xii, 24, 46-47, 63, 234
Vitamin D, xiv, 26, 58, 195-200
Vitamin E, 24, 38, 203
Vitamin synergy, 24

Water, 7, 25, 28, 54, 75, 158, 222
White Bean and Tuna Salad, 86, 106
Wholly Guacamole, 88, 102

Yoga, 143, 146-148, 155-156, 165-172,
    224

Zoe's Split Pea Soup, 85, 100